PAIN

TRAUMA

AND SUICIDE

HOW I OVERCAME

PAIN

TRAUMA

AND SUICIDE

HOW I OVERCAME.

KENNETH GODBOLT III

Dedication

Thank you to all the people who played a role in me becoming the man I am today. To my twin daughters, aka Nanna's, thank you for being the light of my world. I love you and am proud to be your father. My other three E.D.M., you know who you are; thank you for allowing me to play a small role in your life. Dream Big, know I will always be here when you need me. To the youth I encountered at Peoria County Juvenile Detention Center, regardless of how we met, you played a major role in me fighting for mental health and getting back to living my dream.

CONTENT

INTRODUCTION

I woke up one morning and asked myself, *why haven't I been able to achieve mental peace in my life*? When I thought about all that I had been able to accomplish, I realized I was still that broken little boy. I was the first person in my family to graduate high school and college and make it out of my neighborhood. However, parts of my childhood trauma still followed me into my adulthood. No matter how hard I worked, I realized that I had things inside of me that just would not change. I could not change the fact that I still had to sleep with the lights on in my twenties because of the feeling that nothing good happens in the dark. I could not change that when I would have a chronic flashback, I would often think about suicide to stop my brain's madness. It was as if I was living two different lifestyles. The only way to continue to hide it was to pursue success and surround myself with people. I felt as though I could hide my mental health issues behind people-pleasing, but I would grow to learn that you may reach success but will be unable to sustain it if your demons are not dealt with.

I knew that my childhood had caused me more damage than I wanted to admit. I felt that if I acknowledged the pain, it would be a sign of weakness. Growing up, I had never seen a black man seek help for the internal pain they were facing.

Truth be told, I did not want to be the first one because I was afraid of all the backlash I might receive if I opened up. I was also afraid of the work I would have to do to get the results I needed to be the man I knew I could be if I faced my demons. It would take work; it would take me reliving some of my darkest childhood memories. I found myself between a rock and a hard place. On one side, I saw a life of freedom and peace, something that I had never known. On the other side, I saw a version of me who was comfortable with the person I had already become. The young black, mental illness suffering, successful, and broken man people had grown to love, embrace, and admire.

For years, I'd chosen the applause from people over my mental health. It became easier to wear a mask in public and suffer in silence. I'd preached on stages, spoken at schools, college campuses, juvenile detention centers, and prisons, and had the opportunity to travel internationally. I'd seen the impact of how my life story had given others hope. I could not understand how it was possible to give hope to others yet remain hopeless myself. I realized sharing my story was therapeutic for me and offered a sense of freedom for others. Though that seemed to be good and all, I often wondered what it would be like to live in freedom and offer freedom at the same time. If I could accomplish that, life would be so amazing. However, I wondered if that was even possible.

If I wanted to experience the freedom that I knew I could, it would be a long and honest journey, and I would not enjoy the process. I was afraid people would not enjoy the new me, but I had to ask myself if what people thought of me was more important than my own happiness and personal freedom? Was I going to let other people's opinions of me be worth more than me living my God-given purpose? If I wanted to see the changes I desired for this world, I would have to start with myself. I knew it would be a long journey, but it was time to become the real me.

I realized that no matter what I did for the people I loved the most, it would never be good enough; my life only added value when they needed something from me. I walked into the doctor's office and was diagnosed with high blood pressure due to being stressed out from trying to please everyone but myself. It was time for a change. I wanted to know why a person with so much potential and greatness inside of him would spend so much time in unhealthy situations. I needed a reality check; I knew the journey would not be easy, but I had wasted too much of my life running from my calling. I wanted to be happy and enjoy my life. To find peace and freedom, I needed to deal with the unhealthiness in my life. That would require me to take some time away from the routine. Though I did not want to share my story until I'd received the professional help I needed, I did want to share my journey to true freedom.

I struggled with writing this book. I went on Google looking for books written by black men who struggled with mental health. I could not find any, but I knew I was not alone, and I was not the only person working with young black men who desired to know the story of someone struggling with and overcoming mental illness. Writing this book would open up the door for people around the world to acknowledge black mental health. I felt as though people depended on me to tap into my gift and break the ice on a much-needed conversation. That became very apparent to me one day in a conversation with a young man who was about to spend the rest of his life in prison. He had been diagnosed with bipolar disorder early on in his childhood, but because of the stigma associated with his diagnosis, his family refused treatment. One day in a one-on-one conversation, I opened up to him about my struggle with PTSD and how it affected my entire life. I was the first black man to ever open up to him about struggling with a mental disorder. He said, "I really look up to you. I wish I had someone like you in my life before the streets got to me. If I did then, 'my life would have been different." I looked at him and said, "Your life is not over; you can still have an impact." But because he never received the proper care for his mental health, he will now spend the rest of his life in prison. At that moment, I realized how easy it could have been for me to have had a similar outcome.

I don't know why you are reading this book. Maybe it's because something in you resonated with the title, and you said, *Yep, that sounds like me.* Maybe you've heard me speak before and were moved by what you heard. It could be that you have just ended a relationship or marriage and have lost your identity. Maybe you're tired of trying to follow the latest trends in your appearance and social interactions, using outside influences to help you feel accepted instead of just accepting who you really are. You could be the person who used to have a lot of passion for helping others but lost it in the midst of getting hurt and remaining wounded, and now you want to regain your passion again. Maybe someone read this book and decided it would be beneficial for you to read as well, so they bought it for you. Or you have allowed your past to dictate your future, and you're ready to live great and not live like what you have been through. Regardless of why you chose to read this book, you are about to embark on a life-changing journey of a young man who made a brave step to overcome pain, trauma, and suicide.

I'm writing this book because I want to see people physically, mentally, spiritually, and emotionally rich. I am so tired of seeing our world affected by racism, crime, and mental illness because we are afraid to face who we are and what we have become. I imagine what our world would be like if we all lived in our greatness.

It is my hope for people to finally get to the point where they can live free and not allow their pasts to determine their future. Not letting what others think of them to have more value over their lives than the greatness inside of them. I want people to walk away knowing that they were called for a greater purpose. Yes, we all have failed and made mistakes, but our mistakes do not determine whether we live extraordinary lives. If you never get back up, you have allowed your failures and mistakes to win. It would be a sad day at the end of your life if all the people you were supposed to inspire lined up moments before your final breath and said, "I depended on you; I needed to follow your greatness."

This is about you letting go of all the people who have ever hurt you because you know that they have been controlling your life while at the same time enjoying their life. Whatever they did to you that caused you the greatest pain; while you hold on to it, they have long forgotten about it. And if I could be honest, they have also forgotten about you. Yeah, that sucks, but it's the truth. We will dig more into that a little later in the book.

I am about to take you on a journey that has awakened so many things I thought I had dealt with. While writing, I had to take some time away to pause and cry it out. I had to stop and be honest with myself by saying this was still an open wound. I realized that I would have to replace so many lies with the truth about who I was. You will most likely have to do the same, and that's ok. You may have to call some people and have conversations with them for your good. You may have to cut some people off for a while—maybe forever. That's ok as well because now is the time for you to live for yourself.

I don't know about you, but I was tired of waking up depressed and carrying all these burdens when I knew freedom was only one hard choice away—tired of allowing my past to control how I lived my life. Having to realize that I had never been able to live my best life because I have just existed, going through the motions of life. I was making everyone else happy while suffering at the same time. It made no sense, and that is not the way anyone was meant to live.

CHAPTER ONE

TIRED OF RUNNING

"I, this is {redacted}, how may I help you today?"

"I am so tired. I am tired of living. I can't go through the rest of my life like this. I am hurting so bad, and I have been hurting my whole life. Nothing is going to change. I have tried everything. I have tried love, drugs, church, and everything you can find on google. Nothing is working. The only way I will ever have peace is if I am dead. I just have to end my life," I responded. She was so nice on the phone, her voice reminiscent of a nurturing grandmother. She said to me, "Son, I am so sorry you feel this way. What is your name?"

"Ken," I replied.

I was lying in bed, staring at the ceiling with tears running down my face. I began murmuring the words *I'm so tired, I don't want to live anymore.* I grabbed my cell phone and began to scroll through my contacts, looking for someone that I could call and talk to. Sadly, I realized I could not call anyone because I had never let anyone get close to me. Though I had good people around me who genuinely cared, no one knew how I felt and how much I was suffering inside. But I knew I needed someone to talk to, so I picked up the phone and called the crisis hotline.

I grabbed my phone and dialed the hotline, hearing it ring three times. I then heard a stranger's voice on the other end of the line, "Hi, this is…"

"What is your phone number just in case we get disconnected?" I proceeded to give her my phone number and all of the other information she requested.

"Are you in a safe place?" she asked. "No, I am alone right now," I stated.

"Do you have anyone we can call to be there with you?"

"I'm sure I have people who will come, but no one knows that I struggle with this. I'm scared—I'm a leader, and so many people look up to me. This will break their trust and make me look weak."

She replied, "I don't care about anyone else but you right now, and you should only be focused on yourself. I want to help you. So don't talk to me about anyone but you. Now, what's going on?"

"Ma'am, I am so tired. I've been running from things that happened to me as a kid. Things that I have never shared with anyone. I have been having flashbacks of these traumatic experiences since I was five years old. They have been haunting me for years. I have tried everything. I have prayed, I've fasted, I went to healing services at many churches, and I am still haunted almost every day of my life. I've tried sex, I've tried drinking, and I have tried drugs, but I still feel so empty. I walk around with a smile on my face because when I smile, people think I am ok, but in reality, I am not and just need to end it all."

"I don't know you, but I feel you have a lot to offer the world. I'm sorry you are hurting so bad; maybe we need to get you some help. What you be interested in counseling services?" she replied.

I laughed, "Here we go again." "What?"

"So you think walking into some stranger's office and hearing them say, *so how does this make you feel*, and *how does that make you feel* is going to help me? My problems are way too deep for that. I don't know why I called; I keep getting the same answer—counseling, counseling, counseling. I'm a black man; we don't go to counseling. It'd be better if I just killed myself."

Through my entire tirade, she remained polite. "I'm sorry if I offended you; I just want to help."

"No, you did not offend me, I'm just over it, and I am ready to die."

"Ken, do you have a plan?"

"I have many plans," I said. "I think about suicide almost every day."

"Have you ever attempted suicide?"

"Yes, I have tried several times. I tried to shoot myself in the head when I was 15. I took pills when I was

17. I tried to hang myself at 19. I took more pills at 25. I was not successful, but I will make sure I am successful tonight."

"Have you ever been hospitalized?" she asked.

"Yes, I was hospitalized three times, but I lied my way out of them. So, why go to the hospital? All they do is put you on drugs and make you a zombie. And I'm not doing that."

"Thank you for your honesty," she replied. "Ken, I am very concerned for your safety right now and do not feel you should be alone. Do you have a friend that I can call?"

"Yeah, you can call my friend Nelson. I know he will come."

"Ok, what's his number—"

"Wait! I can't—I can't. I'm done talking. I am ready to die. I will finally be at peace."

"Ken, I am sorry you are hurting so bad. Please let me get you help."

"Ma'am, thank you for all your help tonight, but I am ready to go. I'm tired—I'm so tired. I'm going to hang up now."

"Ken, please don't hang up." I hung up the phone.

Imagine struggling just to make it day-to-day and always

getting the same answers. Someone telling you that help is available, and yet nothing is changing in your life. It seems the more you reach out for help, the more you get the people just doing their job to keep you alive but not helping you thrive in life. While I was on the phone with the lady, I could feel she was compassionate, but I also felt nothing was going to change. Though I'd be alive, I would still remain the unhappy, depressed, suicidal young man. That's what led me to hang up the phone and write a suicide note. She had every right to be concerned for me, but her concern could not heal the hurt and pain I felt.

I grabbed a piece of paper, and I did something I had never done before. I wrote a suicide note. In the note, I explained that I knew this would be a shock to many people, that I had chosen to die. I discussed how bad I had been hurting and for how long. I stressed that as they went through life, to pay close attention to the people they loved because I knew I was not the only one who had ever thought about suicide. I closed the letter apologizing to everyone who would show up for my funeral, writing *Do me a favor, don't let other people around you suffer like I did.* I left the letter on the table and walked out of the front door.

As I exited the house, I started walking and saw two police cars circling the neighborhood. I paused, looking like a deer in headlights. If I ran back into the house, they were going to assume I was doing something wrong. I decided to keep walking, and what do you know, they both pulled up next to me. The officer closest to me spoke first.

"Hey man, how are you doing today?"

"Why are you asking me that? I've just left my house, and I'm going on a walk," I said.

"Well, we got a call about a young man who was in distress, and you fit the description."

"Naw, officer. I don't know what you're talking about. I'm just headed to the store to get a drink and some chips."

"What's your name?" he asked, and before I could think of a lie, I responded, "Ken."

"You are the guy we got the call about. What's going on today?" I quickly became very defensive.

"Why you worried about me?"

"We care, man, and just want to help. Look, if we feel you are good, we will call a family member or someone so they can stay with you for the night. I don't know what you are going through, but the lady on the phone was very concerned about you. Let us take you to the hospital to get you some help, man." When he said hospital, I got even angrier.

"I'm not going to no hospital. Them people not going to do anything for me but give me some medication and tell me to talk with someone on the outside. I have already tried that, and it didn't work!"

"Ken, we are just concerned about you. If we had not shown up right this moment, what would you have done tonight?"

I said, "Y'all would have found me dead."

"I would feel more comfortable if you would let us take you in to get evaluated tonight, man. You seem like a good dude, and I don't want you to do anything to hurt yourself."

Because the officer was so nice and calm, I decided to go with him. As I got in the car, I said to him, "Ok. Hey, can you do me a favor? Can you tell the lady on the phone that I'm going to the hospital and that I said thank you?"

He said, "Absolutely," and reached for his handcuffs. "Please don't put the cuffs on me," I said. "I promise I

won't try anything," to which he replied, "OK."

As I sat in the back of the police car that night, I felt like this time would be different for me, but I had no clue how. We arrived at the hospital, where I completed my intake process and was admitted. That night, I could not sleep. I just remember thinking that I was so tired of living like this and that I did not want to continue this cycle. I remembered thinking that one day, I would help other people, but first, I needed to help myself. I promised that night not to fake it this time around but to be real with myself and the doctors. I mean, I knew how the process would go, and I knew how to play their games, and that had gotten me nowhere. The next morning, I met with the doctor for my evaluation.

"Good morning, young man. How are you today?"

I said, "I'm doing good."

"Well, you're not too good if you are here with me. So, I'm going to ask you one more time. How are you doing?"

I said, "Well, life sucks, and I'm ready to just die." "Why do you feel this way?"

"It's a lot, and I don't know if you have enough time to hear me out. So go ahead and give me the medication to zombie me up."

"How can I give you medication if I don't know what's going on with you? You seem agitated today, so we will try this again in the morning." I said, "OK," and walked to my room to lay on the bed and stare at the wall.

While in my room, I can remember thinking to myself, there is something different about this doctor just from how he approached me. I felt as though he was genuine and really wanted to help me. And to be honest, I was struggling with whether or not I really wanted the help. A part of me wanted to give him a chance, but another part of me was afraid he was just doing his job and could not really be this genuine of a person. Especially working in the mental health field.

It was after dinner when I realized that I was alone. I was not surrounded by the people I had tried to please to get to the top. I had no stage to speak on to cover up how I was feeling. It was just me, which was the beginning of seeking peace for myself and not for others. I started asking myself, *how can you be happy and alone? How can you overcome the darkest days of your life and be happy with yourself?* For the first time in my life, I asked the tough questions that could lead me to peace.

Day two.

"Good morning, Ken. How are you today?"

It's my time to see the doctor again. "I'm good," I replied

"Tell me what's good about it?" I said, "I'm still alive."

"Would you still be alive if you were not here?" "I don't know, to tell you the truth."

"I really want to know."

"Well, you will never know because today is the second day; that's 48 hours. I get to go home."

"I'm the doctor, so I get to tell you when you get to leave."

Irate, I said, "You are going to let me go home today, or I am going to go crazy!"

"Well, go crazy then. That's what the hospital for." In my mind, I'm thinking *this dude keeps testing me.* He looked at me and said, "Well, I do not feel comfortable releasing you today, so we will try again in the morning."

I paused on my way out of the office, and I turned to look at him, saying, "Since you kept your word, I will have to keep mine. Turning back around, I walked out of the office and went to my room. I refused everything that day. I did not talk to anyone. I was rude to everyone who tried to talk to me. That night did not go well for anyone, but as I lay in the bed, I realized this doctor would not give up, and I was not going to win. He was not going to let me walk around with my mask on any longer. The stubborn side of me did not want to lose the fight with him. I felt as though the doctor was trying to get to my hurt's depth, and I only wanted to deal with the surface. Never before had I opened up to anyone about my demons and internal darkness. Why would being in the hospital and talking to a man I would never see again be beneficial for me? I was struggling between living with my demons and letting them go. It was as if I was playing tug-o-war with my life and my mental health.

I walked to the door and called the nurse to ask, "How long can they keep me in here?" She looked at my chart and said, "Your insurance will cover 30 days and will cover longer if we need them too." I started to walk off when she said, "We can get a court order for you to stay longer if the doctor does not think you are fit to leave. By the way, if you think you're going to win with this doctor, you won't. He's just that good. In the end, he will win."

I did not want to hear that. I walked away, deciding to give up. I had met my match. My pride was not happy, but my soul felt at peace. I arrived at my room, and all I could think was that the nurse was right. This doctor was not going to let me walk out of here the same. No matter how hard I pushed him or fought him, he had seen and worked with people like me before and had way more experience. And after two days, he had not backed down, nor had he given up on helping me. I knew I would not win this fight, admitting it was a fight I *needed* to lose. What I would gain from losing this battle was more important and essential to the life I wanted. I was still fighting to win a battle I'd been losing my entire life. My mental health had caused more damage to me and others than I would have liked to admit.

Day three.

"Good morning, Ken." "Good morning, Doc."

"How are you doing today?"

"I'm not doing too good. First, I want to apologize to you for being rude and giving you a hard time."

"No apology needed; I'm used to it." I thought to myself, *man, this dude is cocky*. He continued, "Now, let's get started. I want to know what's going on with you."

I said, "Man, I had a rough life. I've seen some things I did not want to see. I have experienced things that a child should never have had to experience. It has been tormenting me for years. I have frequent flashbacks; the images play in my mind as if I'm watching a movie. I'm tired of dealing with it. I'm tired of running from it. I don't know how to deal with this, so I feel like it's better to die. I'm just tired."

"I see you have a history of suicidal ideation." "Yeah, you can say that."

"How has that worked out for you?"

"Well, obviously, I've been unsuccessful." "What did the other doctors say to you.?

"They told me I was bipolar and just needed medications."

The doctor laughed. "I see why you don't trust us.

You are not bipolar. You have PTSD, son." "What is that, Doc?"

"It's when you go through something traumatic, and it haunts you, affecting your life if not dealt with. When was your first experience?"

I told him I was very young, like my second year of kindergarten or first grade.

"You have been suffering for a very long time. I am shocked that you have made it this far. On the first day I met you, I went home and could not sleep. I said, 'why is this kid here?' I told my wife that I had a tough one on my hands. There's something about this kid."

"Thanks, doc," with tears in my eyes, I asked, "Can you really help me?"

"Yes, but you will have to do most of the work." "I will work because I am so tired of suffering."

"I am going to keep you here for a few more days, and we are going to work on getting you healthy. You have a lot of potential. You are a special kid."

Never in my wildest dream did I think I would find the help I needed in the hospital. For the next few days, the Doc and I met up and talked. I was feeling so good; I felt like I could take on the world again. I felt hope for the first time in my life. But my heart dropped when the nurse came and said it was time for me to be discharged. I met with the doctor for the last time, and he was very encouraging. He said he believed I could do it out there. I did not believe him; I knew a world that did not care about what I had gone through. I was going to a place with no support system. I just felt really nervous and terrified.

All the work I'd put in at the hospital would last for about a year and a half when I would find myself in yet another broken place—this time, I did something totally different. I did not think about killing myself; I decided that I was going to seek therapy. I went into the therapist's office and said, "Look, I'm broken, and I'm tired. I don't want to kill myself like the other times. I have a reason to live. I want to live my passions, but first, I need to deal with my heart. My past has haunted me my entire life, and I'm ready to do whatever I need to get healthy."

That day in her office, I told her my whole life story and how much pain I was in. I told her that I was tired of running and wanted to know what it was like to live a healthy lifestyle. In the end, she looked at me and said, "You have a lot going on, so we will deal with one issue at a time. I believe we can get you to the place where you are enjoying life."

CHAPTER TWO

ACKNOWLEDGING THE PAIN AND TRAUMA

Tap, Tap, Tap.

That was the sound I heard on the window that night. It wasn't the first time I'd heard that sound, though. I was used to hearing the sound several times during the week. On this particular night, I wished I would have never heard that tapping sound. It was my mother's boyfriend. He and my grandmother did not get along, so my mom would sneak him into the house late at night. My mother would do her normal routine, then she would grab the door and place it in the doorway. The door was off the hinges as a result of a domestic dispute. She would then slide the dresser by the door so that no one could come into the room. Then, she would open the window, and he would climb into the room. I would usually grab my blanket and make a pallet on the floor, but that would not be the case that night.

When he entered the room that night, he was irate. They started to argue, cussing and yelling at each other. He seemed to be upset that my mother had male friends, and he assumed she was cheating on him. They went from yelling and screaming to him beating her. I remembered every slap and every punch. I remember my mom making *ooh* and *ouch* sounds every time he hit her. She was crying and begging him to stop, but he would not. I was so scared and afraid and begged him to stop, but he looked at me with a smile on his face and told me to shut up. I started to cry when he looked at me and told me to *shut up and stop crying like a little sissy. Stop acting like a little girl*. My tears of sadness turned to tears of rage and anger that night. All I could think about was killing him one day.

After he stopped beating my mom, he grabbed what appeared to be gasoline, a red rag, and a green lighter. He began to strike the lighter repeatedly, laughing, making jokes about killing us. He even said *y'all are going to die tonight*. I remember my mother begging and pleading with him to stop, but he continued to laugh, all while playing with the lighter. *I hope y'all ready to die tonight*. My mom continued to beg him to stop; she said *I will do whatever you want me to do. Just stop. Please don't hurt us*, but he continued making threats. This seemed to be a game to him. He knew he could overpower us but what he did not know was that he was turning a little boy into a monster.

As they continued to argue, he revealed that he was upset because he believed that my mother did not want to be with him anymore. He stated that if he could not have her, then no one else could. Even if that meant my mother dying along with the rest of us. My mother pleaded that she did want to be with him and no one else. It was as if she had to choose between our lives or remaining in an abusive relationship. After seeing that she was serious, he placed the lighter, gasoline, and rag on the dresser. He stated *you're mine, and no one else's*, and my mother shook her head yes. They embraced each other and laid down in the bed, deciding to have intimate relations, while I grabbed my blanket and made my pallet on the floor, afraid to go to sleep. I was used to the intimacy and the beating, but what happened tonight was more traumatizing than anything I had ever encountered before. I saw a man threaten to kill a mom and a son over jealousy and still win over the heart of the mom, who was supposed to protect her son first.

While they kissed and made out, all I could do was cry as I laid awake unable to sleep. All I could see was his face, hearing his threats, his punches as he hit my mom, all while the tears of anger and rage ran down my face. I knew that as a little boy, I could not do anything to hurt him. Though he was skinny, he stood over 6'6. My little frame would cause him no damage. Though I could not do anything that night, I knew one day I would grow up, and I would have my opportunity. I made a vow that night to be a murderer—I was going to kill him when I got older. He was going to have to pay for what he did to us on that day. I imagined having a gun in my hand, shooting him several times in the face. *You remember that little boy who you called a sissy for crying? Well, now I'm old enough to defend myself.* I remembered looking at my mom and making a vow that I would never let another man beat her ever again. Any man that put his hands on my mother would be killed as well. All I could remember was laying down that night and silently crying myself to sleep. While the man I vowed to kill and the mother I vowed to protect slept in the same bed cuddled together as lovers.

The next morning my mother woke me up for school, and I completed my morning routine. As I got ready to leave, my mother grabbed me and told me not to tell anyone about what had happened last night. My whole body went numb as I said, "ok." I grabbed my backpack and started my walk to school. When I got to the corner, my mother's boyfriend was right there. I was so scared I could hear my heart pounding. He told me to come here, and when I walked over to him, he said, "You better not say anything about what happened last night." I looked at him and said, "ok." That was one of the hardest walks to school I had ever had. I wanted to cry, but I couldn't. I could not seem to process what had happened on my own, yet I had no one that I could process it with. I was afraid that if I shared what happened with anyone, I would be putting my mother and my life in jeopardy. The consequences of me telling someone felt greater than me freeing myself of the pain I was feeling. I learned some dangerous lessons that day. I learned to internalize my feelings and my emotions and to never, ever express my pain. If an adult hurt me, don't say a word. And that's exactly what I did. I shared that night with no one. I closed my eyes as if nothing ever happened.

Fast forward a few months, I would be molested by a female family member. This would not be a one-time incident but would happen several times over a small time frame. She would not be the only one to molest me—it would happen again, a total of three different females and multiple encounters. And they all said the same thing after molesting me that my mother and her boyfriend said to me. *Don't tell anyone about what just happened; keep it our little secret.* When those words were said to me, I knew at that moment whatever had just happened to me was wrong. But again, I did not know how to deal with it or have anyone to talk to. Instead, I just put my head down and attempted to go through life, blocking the images out of my head.

The more I attempted to block the pain, the angrier I became. School seemed to be the best place for me to express my anger. I spent days in the principal's office, school suspensions, and went through many alternative programs, but none of them worked. I was a huge distraction for the other kids learning around me, and I gave my teachers hell. But the hell I gave them and the other students could not compare to the emotional turmoil I was feeling inside. Though they attempted to provide me with the help I needed, the pain was too deep. I had no idea how to express it.

When I was in the third grade, I thought I had found help for my trauma. Our school guidance counselor came into our classroom and spoke to our class about abuse. As she began to speak, her first topic was sexual abuse. I sat there in my chair and replayed all the incidents I'd had with the three females who'd molested me. I remember thinking to myself, I knew something was not right, and what happened to me should not have been going on. I realized that I had been sexually abused. She then continued to share about domestic abuse, parent-to-parent, and parent-to-child. I began to replay that night my mom's boyfriend beat her and threatened to kill us. She closed her presentation with, "If you have ever experienced any of these types of abuse, my office is always open to talk. I promise I will do whatever I can to help." I was sitting in that chair holding back the tears, scared. But I kept thinking about the two words she said *help* and *safety*. I knew I needed help, as the abuse and pain were eating away at me every day and every night. I also wanted to feel safe; I wanted to know what it was like to be protected and free from pain and trauma. I wanted someone to help me see that I had hope and that I would be okay. Something I had never felt or experienced throughout any of my traumatic encounters.

I remember wondering to myself what I should do at that moment. A part of me thought the right thing to do was talk to her about everything because she would help me. Then I would remember all the people who caused the pain had told me not to tell anyone about what happened. My heart was pounding, and I was afraid, but I decided to be a brave young man. I walked into her office and sat in her chair. I asked her if I could talk with her, and she said sure. I told her, "I have experienced a lot of the things you talked about today."

She said, "Please tell me what happened." I told her I'd been sexually abused, and I'd witnessed the fighting she talked about. I proceeded to go into the details of my mom's boyfriend beating her and threatening to kill us. I relived these pains every day of my life, and as I talked, she wrote down everything. After I finished speaking, she got up and left the room. She came back with a snack and a drink. It was almost as if I was in a police interrogation room.

About 15 minutes later, my grandmother and her boyfriend walked through the doors. I remember looking scared and afraid because I was very shocked to see them. At the same time, I knew seeing them was not good for me. They left me in the room alone, and the adults went somewhere else to talk. When they came back into the room, I could see the anger on their faces. My guidance counselor then told me I was being checked out for the day. I stared at her, us both locking eyes. I walked away thinking, *I thought you were going to help me?* My grandmother just screamed and yelled at me the whole way home.

"Why the hell did you tell them people that? You want them to take you away? The next time you pull this stunt, I'm going to let them take you."

Her boyfriend interjected on a yell, "I want to know why he would say something like that! We need to get to the bottom of why he said what he said!"

"I don't give a damn why he said that. I don't want them people in my face with this bull. You know how this makes us look?" she said.

"Something had to happen for him to say that. A child would not just make something up like that. I want to know why." At that moment, I zoned out as they continued to argue.

When I got home, my grandmother screamed, "Go to the room, and don't you come out!" So, I walked to the room and laid on the bed. I was thinking to myself, is this why they told me not to say anything? Were they trying to protect themselves, or did they know no one would believe me, and it was a waste of time to even talk about it? I heard the door open, and when I looked up, there was my uncle standing there with a belt. He had this angry look on his face and began to beat me with the belt.

"What the hell did you tell them people?! Don't you ever tell them white folks what goes on in this house!" I remembered every hit, and with every strike of his belt, it was more confirmation that no matter what happened to me in life, I was safer just enduring the pain and not talking about it. From that day on, I decided that I would walk through this life, keeping my pain, abuse, and trauma to myself.

I used to pray that it would all fade away one day, and the memories of the incidents would leave my mind for good. That would be far from reality. For years and years, I battled with depression and suicide, wishing and hoping the pain would stop. Going through life as wounded as I was would only lead me to many situations that added to my pain. We have all heard this saying before, *Hurt people, hurt people.* By not dealing with my own issues, I knew the people around me were not dealing with their issues either. So, the hurt just continued throughout life.

I would become another young black teen who would go through life affected by his trauma. Wearing a mask of toughness to prove nothing affected me while all along dying inside. And because of my trauma, I would run the risk of either dying from unresolved issues or spending my life in prison. It would be assumed that I'd become a womanizer with multiple kids and multiple baby mothers, all while playing hard in the streets hustling. In reality, all I really wanted was to be free from the pain I had to witness and experience for years. The freedom I'd likely never know because the men who looked like me said I was soft if I allowed my pain and trauma to affect who I would become.

Society told me that I needed to just get over it because everybody goes through something. All you had to do was try hard, and good things would happen for you. I wish that had been the truth. No matter how hard I tried, the flashbacks were real and never got easier. My emotions continued to get the best of me because I never learned how to process my pain. I will tell you that you can never become the person you want until you deal with the hurt inside of you. Age does not heal, time does not heal, and ignoring does not heal. Just like age does not mean maturity, time does not equal growth and maturity. But when I decided to heal the little boy in me, that's was when change and growth began to happen. And that's what I did the day I looked in the mirror and decided that I was ready to heal the little boy inside of this 6'2, 265-pound man.

CHAPTER THREE

ABANDONMENT

As a child, I longed for my mother's love and affection, but I could not receive it due to her drug addiction, sickness, and unhealthy relationships. Prior to her death, I could count on one hand the times she ever told me that she loved me. Due to this, my love tank was empty most of my life, and I struggled with abandonment issues. If my own mother could not love and protect me, why would anyone else in the world want to? This would leave me with trust issues, and I would go through the majority of my life never trusting anyone. To protect my heart from ever feeling that feeling again, I began to build a wall around my heart, never allowing myself to feel what real love was supposed to feel like.

I was born on March 12, 1983, to teenage parents. My father was very upset with my mother the day I was brought home from the hospital. In his anger and pain, he cut her with a machete. My mother would be left with three visible scars, one on her forehead, her forearm, and one on the back of her leg, which she received trying to get away. My mother survived the attack, and my father was later arrested and taken to jail. After hearing this story, I have often wondered if that was a sign that my life would be full of challenges and dark days. Though I did not witness what happened, I believe some of my mother's resentment towards my father played a role in how she treated me as an infant. I mean, think about it, this happened on the first day I came home from the hospital.

I don't remember much about my relationship with my mother during my younger years. But I do remember the morning I heard a hard knock on the door. My house was being raided by the police. *Boom! Boom! Boom!* The door flew open as the police forced everyone to the ground. Guns were pointed at everyone in the house, including me, as I laid in the lap of one of my uncles, and every adult in the house would be placed in handcuffs and arrested. The police officers tore through our house, ripping it apart as they searched for drugs. The police took every adult to jail, except my grandmother. I watched my mom be placed into the police car as I cried and screamed for them to let her go. I stood in the driveway as they drove off with my mother. She was taken to jail for the sale and delivery of crack cocaine. That day, I developed a hatred for police officers, as I felt they stole my mother from me.

The next time I saw her was when my grandmother took me to the prison to visit. I remember having to walk through these gates to a picnic table where we waited for her to come out. She came out with her blue scrub-like outfit on, and my face lit up. I sat in her lap as we laughed, played, and talked. What felt like a few minutes later, the guards came and took my mother away. I cried myself to sleep every time we had to leave. I could not understand why the police would take my mom away from me and put her in that place. I felt that every time I would get close to her or feel her affection, it would instantly be taken away and this would become the theme of our relationship from a young age into my adolescence.

At that time in my life, I did not know that they would have to let her go one day, but eventually, they did. That day she was released will always be a memory engraved inside my head. I was walking home from school, and I could see her standing in the driveway of our home, with a t-shirt and green army pants on. I ran so fast down the road to get to her and gave her the biggest hug ever. Finally, my mother was home, and no one would ever take her away again. Man, that was the best feeling and greatest moment as a kid to have your mother home. Life was going to be so great. And though it was great for the moment, I did not get to enjoy it as long as I would have liked to. It would be very shortlived, and I would be headed to my darkest of days.

Shortly after being released from prison, my mother would be introduced to using *crack*, a drug that had been destroying the black community through the 1980s well into the 1990s, and it is still very prevalent today. She would struggle with addiction until she passed away in the summer of 2005. This drug changed my mother for the worse. It seemed she would do whatever it took to get it, and it became her priority, while at the same time, my siblings and I were fighting for her attention. At that time in my life, I could not understand the power of addiction. I just felt as though her drug fix was more important than her children.

Once she was addicted to drugs, I never felt close to her again in my childhood. I never again embraced her like I did the day she came home from prison. I grew distant from her, unable to feel loved and nurtured by her. Because she was ashamed, my mother would never come to any school functions or sports activities. I used to look up in the stands and wish she were there watching me. My mother's struggle with addiction affected a lot of my lack of mental development as a child. It led me to struggle with emotional and behavioral challenges. I was placed in an emotional handicap EH class for behavioral issues at an early age. I struggled with communicating with others; the only way I communicated was through outbursts of violence. I hated rules and routines because I knew they would never stay the same, and our living in poverty prevented us from having any kind of stability or structure.

My mother would be hit with yet another blow in my adolescent years when she was diagnosed with AIDS. She had gone to the clinic to get tested, and the doctors called to share her test results. The day she found out was tortuous, she walked up and down the street screaming and crying, "No! No! No! No!" She eventually went into the house and locked herself in the bedroom, continuing to scream and cry. I wanted to know what was wrong with her, but I could not get an answer. I wanted to help her, but I had no idea how to do so or what would come next. I just knew that whatever news she had gotten was not good. After a few days of withdrawing from the family, she sat me down and had a conversation. She said, "Son, I'm dying. I have a sickness, and not many people make it that long. Son—I have AIDS." I had no idea what that was because it was still a new thing around that time. But watching how everyone treated us after she was diagnosed, it became apparent that it was bad, scary, and highly infectious. Though my mother had not died yet, people treated her as if she was the walking dead.

Shortly after, we were forced to move out of my grandmother's house because of her sickness. I was scared and afraid, but there was a part of me that did not want to leave my mother alone. I knew she was hurting from her sickness, and I did not want to leave her all alone. For the next year and a half, we spent our lives in and out of different people's homes. The majority of the places we stayed in were drug houses. As a kid, I tried to block everything out, but I could not help what I was witnessing. Watching the drug addicts get high and fill the rooms with crack smoke, drug dealers fighting with the addicts for not paying them, and women selling themselves for drugs took a toll. Though it was challenging, I knew this was all I had at the time, and it was better than the other alternative of not having any place to go at all. On the nights we could not find a place to stay, we would sneak and stay at my grandmother's house. Her house was behind a railroad track, so we would take the tracks instead of the streets so no one would see us. My mom would open the window, I would climb in, and she'd climb in after me. Then we would sleep for a few hours and leave very early the next morning so that no one knew we were there.

My sisters and my brother lived with relatives in the same neighborhood. My sisters' grandmother opened her home to my mother and me. Mary became my grandmother and took me into her home, loving me as her own. I felt safe and whole at her home because I knew she would protect us. The idea of knowing I had a stable home and a place to lay my head at night became my security. That would only last a short while, as I could not follow the rules and wanted to do things my own way. I was still getting into trouble at school and causing problems. I resented my sisters who lived there with me because I felt they did not have to go through the same things I had to go through. I really wanted stability and good home life. But I did everything I could to ruin it. I was comfortable living from house to house.

I would continue this cycle for a few years until I met a friend by the name of Kenneth. Yeah, we shared the same first name, and we were both named after our fathers. We developed a great relationship, and I spent a lot of my weekends over at his house. They were dropping me off home one day and realized that I did not have lights or water. My mother and my friend's mom, Denise, talked, and they both agreed it would be better for me to move in with them until my mother got on her feet. Denise did not judge my mother for her struggles but wanted to give me a chance at a better life. That would again be short-lived due to my behavior issues at school. Being that KK and I had the same name. He was getting in trouble because the school was calling for Kenneth. The Kenneth they were speaking of was me. I could not stay out of trouble. I was fighting, cussing out teachers, and being rebellious. Denise sat me down and stated that she loved me but could not allow me to set a bad example for KK. At that time, I did not understand, but I get it now. I was given several opportunities to change, but I continued to get in trouble. She had no choice but to send me back to my neighborhood with my mother.

Though I had many people around me that wanted the best for me, I could not receive it. I couldn't fault Mary or Denise because they did not know the level of pain and hurt I was dealing with. Yet, I believed they would have helped me get the help I needed.

Where was my father throughout all of the pain? That's a great question. It was probably better for him not to be around at that time of my life. My father would only add to the wall of broken hearts from my adolescent years. I remember he would call me on Thursday nights, and the phone would ring.

"Hello?"

"Can I speak with Yogi?" "Yeah, who is this?"

"It's his daddy," then the phone would be passed to me.

"Hey, dad!" excitement spreading over my face.

"You have your bag packed? I'm coming to get you tomorrow after work."

"OK, Dad," I'd hang up the phone and grab my grandmother's old blue suitcase that looked like a miniature coffin. I would pack my bag and have it ready to go even though I knew deep down I would probably be disappointed. But I was a kid, so I was so excited. For little boys, there's nothing you want more than to spend time with your father. Those Fridays at school, I would watch the clock waiting to go home because I knew it was daddy's weekend.

After school, I would run home, put my suitcase by the

front door to be ready for my father when he came and got me. No matter how many times he had failed in the past, I just knew this would be the time he would come. Every time I would get my hopes up, and he would fail. I remember sitting by the door, angry that my dad did not want to spend time with me. What did I ever do to him for him not to be in my life? My heart grew colder towards him with every failed attempt, which would soon turn into hatred and anger.

He knew my mom was struggling with drugs and battling addiction. He knew that I would sleep in homes without food and lights while he was married with kids and had an extra bedroom in his house. He would have been able to give me a better life than the life I was living and would have been able to help me avoid many of the dark nights I had faced. With every opportunity he had to become my hero, he just added to the pain I would have to endure.

My mom would often threaten to call my dad when I got into trouble. That would be the only time he wanted to become a "hero." I would blurt out, "Call him; he ain't gon' do nothing to me. He can't even show up when he's supposed to." She would tell me that he was going to whoop me, and my response was always that, "If he hits me, I'm going to hit him back. He's not my dad but a sperm donor." If he could hit me, he could have shown up when he said he would. He had no problem showing up to my court dates and discipline meetings at school, though.

One day I got into a fight at school and was suspended. My mother decided to call my dad and let him know that I was in trouble. That day he stopped whatever he was doing and made a special trip to my house. I was outside playing football with my friends and saw his car pull up. He knew I saw him, but I ignored him. He yelled, "Get you but over right now." I continued to act as if I did not hear what he was saying. He walked over and grabbed my arm, but I yanked away from him.

"Don't you put your hands on me ever again," I said, turning away, and he proceeded to smack me in the arm. I turned around and looked him in his face, and repeated, "Don't you ever put your hands on me again, or we are fighting." Then, I walked away. He continued to call out to me but knew I was too angry to have a conversation.

That day was very pivotal in my relationship with my father. I knew that he could tell I was hurting and had lost all respect for him as my father. But in the back of my mind, I knew that if I ever wanted to see him, all I had to do was get into trouble. I knew then that he would never show up to my award ceremonies or sports games, but he would gladly show up to all my court dates, conferences, and probation meetings. So, at that time in my life, getting into trouble became a normal routine. It was the only way that I could see my father.

I wanted him to save me. I wanted him to be the

superman who came in and saved the day, rescuing me from my troubles. That day would never come for me. Instead, I lost another parent to addiction. My father was what people called a "functioning alcoholic." He started and ended his day with a beer in his hand. The only way I thought I would be able to go through life was to act as if he did not exist to protect my heart. I don't have many memories of him as a child, and the ones I do have are not good. No matter what, I still spent most of my days longing and wishing I knew what it was like to grow up feeling love and affection from a father.

Though I was not alone, I grew up feeling empty of love and affection and abandoned, which has affected how I view relationships with other people. I never allowed myself to get too close, and when I did, it was only close enough to where it would not hurt me if I had to let them go. Due to the hurt I felt from my parents, the moment I felt I was experiencing anything related to what I did as a child, I would immediately go into what I called the "turtle complex," like when a turtle senses danger and immediately goes into their shell to hide from the danger, or in my case, familiar behavior.

Later, after going through the healing process, it was no wonder that most of my relationships were toxic. From birth, my relationship with my parents set the foundation for toxicity to grow. I remember one particular relationship where I was kicked out of the house several times and had to sleep in rest areas and hotels. Though I would go back several times, I knew I was done the first time I had been asked to leave, as it made me relive those moments as a child, which were still affecting me in my adulthood. I lived in my shell for the remaining part of the relationship, doing what I had to do for a place to stay. The disfunction did not bother me, as I was comfortable in my shell. I'd become comfortable being abandoned.

CHAPTER FOUR

UNDIAGNOSED

I fought long and hard with whether I should write this chapter or not, but I made a promise to myself that if I was going to write this book, I wanted to be as open and as honest as possible with my readers. Almost every morning that I woke up, I would utter the phrase, *I can't do this anymore.* I would often think about suicide, wanting my life to be over. I was tired of hurting and did not feel I would ever get to live life with some relief. It's not that I wanted to physically die, but I wanted the pain to die, and if the pain would not die, the only way I felt I could stop it was to kill myself. This started at the age of eight years old. I was very upset with my family because I always felt like the black sheep, and one day I'd had enough. After arguing with them, I told everyone that I was going to jump in front of a train. At that moment, I thought they would have some compassion and realize something was going on with me. But I got the opposite reaction. They started laughing, called me a crazy bastard, and made a joke out of how I was feeling that day. That experience was the first time that I associated how I was feeling with being crazy. Even at that young age, I knew that being crazy was not a good thing. I knew it to be the young lady down the road who would sit on her porch and make funny noises as she rocked back and forth in her rocking chair. It was the people I would see walking down the street talking to themselves or how the movies portrayed people in straitjackets getting shots to help them calm down. I got freaked out by those comparisons, and that would spare my life that day because if I jumped in front of the train, I would be remembered as the kid who was crazy.

Though it kept me from committing suicide, it did not stop me from thinking about it. It did not ease the pain that I felt every day. When I was fifteen, I attempted suicide for the first time in my life. I felt at that time when everything was going wrong, I could not deal with the pressure. It was the first time I grew tired of always feeling like I had to keep it all together. That night, I took a loaded pistol and put it to my head. I squeeze the trigger, and nothing happened. I walked outside and screamed and yelled, "I can't do this anymore! I don't want to live!" One of my childhood friends ran outside to try and help me. He was confused and scared because he had never seen me act like this. I grabbed him and stated, "I can't even kill myself right." I told him not to tell anyone about what I'd done. He was scared but told me that I better not do anything like that again. I was so angry and wanted to die; I was over life. Nothing was going right. I wasn't in school, my home life was a mess, and I really did not have anything to live for.

Two years later, I would attempt suicide a second time, but this would lead me to my first hospital visit. It was close to the holidays, and I found myself alone for Christmas. I'd heard that people who struggled with mental illness took the holidays extremely hard. My girlfriend and I were also going through a little high school lovers quarrel, and we ended up breaking up. A part of me was kind of excited because I did not have to buy her a gift, but then I was upset because I thought I was in love. I walked through the house, trying to find a way to be positive, but I couldn't. I was really desperate for a reason to live, but I could not find one at the time. I went into my cabinet and grabbed two different bottles of pills and took them all. I called one of my friends and told him what I did. He immediately came to my house, grabbed me, and took me to the hospital. When I arrived at the hospital, they told me that I would be admitted and placed a security guard by my door. I looked up and saw it was a friend of our family's, named Pastor Joe. At that moment, I had all types of feelings going through my body at this time. I felt like my secret was out, and he was going to inform my family members of my struggles. I was not at the place in my life where I wanted them to know. I thought since he was a pastor, he would reach out to me and try and give me some spiritual guidance outside of the hospital. Most of all, I felt that my secret struggle with mental health was exposed. I remained nervous because I didn't know if he would expose it or not. He looked at me and asked how I was doing but never said anything to my family or me. To this day, he has never asked me about anything. The next morning the doctor came in to do an evaluation, and I told him everything he wanted to hear so I could go home. He decided to keep me one more day and released me the day after. I wish I could tell you that experience was good, but it was a joke. Not because of the doctor but more because I was not honest with my feelings and well-being. I continued on my journey of unstable living with no relief.

I went to a private school during this time, so we would have chapel every week. I would sit in the chapel and tune out whatever the speaker was saying. But one day, they brought a group of speakers in from a program called "teen challenge," and it really rocked me. These were a group of men who had overcome drug addiction and were living life in a powerful way. One of the men who was speaking said, no matter what you are going through in your life, God can fix it. He saved me from a long life of drug addiction. He loves you right where you are at." I remember the day I broke down in chapel service. I needed to be fixed, and I was willing to try anything at that point. The speaker said, "If you want God to fix your life, ask him to forgive you of your sins and come into your heart. He will do it." I followed what he said, and it felt really good.

I was impacted by that moment and decided that I wanted to give up my dreams of playing basketball to become a preacher. For the next two years, I did not miss a church service; any day the doors were open, I was there. When it came to picking a college, I wanted to go to a Christian university and study ministry, and that's what I did. I chose to attend Southeastern University in Lakeland, Florida. I wanted to get my degree so that I could go out and save the world. I went to church at least five days a week. One day, one of my friends in college told me I was a church junkie. He told me I was there every time the doors opened, and he was right. I felt that if I wanted to stay sane, I needed to be in a church as often as possible.

I had to be in church every time the doors opened because, when I did not go to church, I had a hard time coping with life. I wanted to get in the service and hear the music because it gave me a sense of peace. But honestly, during my time in college, my faith was like a roller coaster. I was still unbalanced and unhealthy. I struggled a lot with whether I should stay in college or go back home and run the streets. I felt guilty because I was the first person in my family to attend college, and my family back home was suffering. Many of my childhood friends got arrested and sentenced to prison. Others were using heavy drugs and overdosing, throwing their lives away. I felt that if I were to go home, I would have stopped some of them. A couple friends I was close to were murdered during this time, which made me feel as though I had escaped death, but just barely. I had several suicide attempts in college while in my dorm room, but I was the young man who had dreams to save the world when I left the room. It was apparent to many that I had deep issues, but I walked around wearing a mask.

After graduating college, I got married and took a job as a youth pastor at an amazing church in Tampa, FL. This was an amazing time; the staff I worked with was amazing, and I was able to work with at-risk teenagers. I completed my first Christian hip-hop album called "True Freedom," but I was far from free. During that time, my mask was still on because what was happening in my home life did not match the life that I portrayed from the pulpit to the people I was leading. Two unhealthy people battled their own mental illnesses, loving God but hating each other and themselves. I wanted to escape, to get out, but I was afraid because of the stigma that would come with divorce. So I stayed. I was told to pray and fast, so I did. I was told to go to counseling, and I did that. Finally, one day I'd had enough and said this was it, the final time. I had to be successful with suicide. Not even church or Jesus could fix me.

I left the house with a bottle full of pills and drove around the Tampa area. I drove to a gas station and walked in to buy a bottle of water to take the pills with. I walked to the counter, and the cashier asked me how I was doing? I told her not good and that I was on my way to kill myself. I handed her the letter where I'd written my ex-wife's number and told her to call it to let them know I was going to kill myself. I would be dead by the time someone found me. I walked out of the store, sat in my car, and took the whole bottle of pills. I then drove to a local park and sat in the car. I thought it was actually over for me this time. I became very light-headed as my heart pounded heavily in my chest. Out of all the times I wanted to die, this was the first time I'd had thoughts of wanting to live. But I thought it was too late. At that moment, I decided to pray, telling God I didn't want to die; I wanted the pain to die. A few minutes later, I threw up the pills I'd taken and was found five minutes later, alive. I was taken to the hospital, where I actually found the doctor that allowed me to find hope to begin the healing process.

I want to be clear; I don't blame God for my battles with suicide. I take full responsibility for all of my actions and how my attempts have affected the people I was around. I have learned over time that mental illness does not discriminate. It does not care about your religion, race, age, gender, sexuality, or social status. So for me, to blame anyone for specific things would give you an inaccurate view of the struggle that I went through. However, I believe there were signs that I'd given others, warning signs that even I'd ignored.

My mental health was not the only thing affected. My physical health was as well. I ended up in the hospital several times one month, and some of those times would cause me to have to be admitted. In many of those cases, the doctors could not find anything wrong with me. One particular hospital visit, the doctor noticed I had a hernia, and they decided I would need surgery. The doctor said during the surgery, they would also explore my other organs. The next day when the doctor came to visit me, he stated that I had the best set of organs he had seen in a long time and that I should look into some counseling, to deal with my real health issue. He stated that he believed my health issues were caused by my mental state more than my physical. He asked if my home life was good, to which I told him yes. But the reality was that it was not. I was suppressing what was going on at the time, which had started to affect my mental health.

You may be wondering why I shared this chapter with you. I shared this for two reasons. One, so you could get a real-life account of what it looks like to be unhealthy, for you to get a clear picture of what it's like for some people to live with trauma and how hard it is for them to survive day-to-day. People are suffering, and if they share they are struggling to live, take it seriously and try to get them the help they need. It can be tougher than you think and sometimes hard to understand what's going on with them. If they can't understand it, what makes you think you will understand their suffering? Even in your understanding, you may not help them reach the same level of understanding. I also shared this chapter for the person whose struggles may resemble my own and have lived this way for a long time. I want you to know that there is hope, and you can overcome this. Yes, you will have to work at it, and it won't be easy, but the life you can live after you have faced your pain can be pretty enjoyable. Continue to push for your freedom, and don't give up.

This book is only a small glimpse of what day-to-day life was like for me during this process. I wish there was time to walk you through everything and every situation. I was mentally and physically tired most of my life, and when I hear people say that some have taken the easy way out, well, I do not consider living your life wanting to die every day as an easy life. There is always hope, but our world can be judgmental that many people are afraid to seek the help they need. I was only the right diagnosis away from living a balanced and healthy life. Just imagine if I would have found this hope earlier in my life. What if I would have successfully committed suicide and could have been helped with just a diagnosis?

We must begin to tear down the stereotypes of what it

means to be diagnosed with a mental illness and normalize the importance of getting help. Many people today are undiagnosed and would benefit from knowing the reason(s) why they feel the way they do. They are not crazy; they have a medical issue that can be treated. We would never tell a person with diabetes to eat whatever they wanted and live life like a person with-out diabetes. We would encourage them to take their insulin and watch what they eat. Mental illness needs to become just as important as diabetes, and maybe we could see a healthier world. It feels like more people die every year because of mental illnesses, and yet people are still undiagnosed and suffering when we have the tools to help. We need more people to be diagnosed instead of dying because they have suffered from being undiagnosed.

CHAPTER FIVE

UNLOVED

One key component to the suffering I went through was I never built real relationships with other people. Every relationship I had was superficial and had no substance. I never gave myself the chance to experience real and genuine friendships. Yet, I didn't know how to because my walls were up so high. The moment I allowed someone to get close to me, they would eventually hurt me. Why would I believe that people could care about me when the two people that were supposed to love me the most had caused me the most pain and hurt? Here I was, in my late twenties, and I'd never had the opportunity to experience true intimacy with anyone.

When I think about friendships, there are two people who come to mind. The first person is a man named Nelson. I met Nelson in college, and we hit it off on the very first day we met. He was a real and genuine dude, and I can honestly say he did everything in his power to make sure I was good. When I was hurting, he hurt with me. The times I had to be admitted to the hospital, he was there with his arms wide open and did not judge me. When my mother passed away, he and his wife drove 3 hours to be with me at the funeral. When I lost everything, he opened his home and gave me a job to get back on my feet. Anytime I called his phone for anything, he would do whatever he could for me with no hesitation. I had spurts in my life where I was able to give that back to him, but I could not do it consistently. If I can be honest, I feel like I broke him as a man several times throughout our friendship. Though his love for me was pure, I could not see it because I was still looking through a broken lens.

I would say the next person I was close with was Martin. He was a drummer in our church, and his wife worked with me at the church. Martin and I would talk all the time and spend a lot of our time fishing and eating. There was never a time when we were together that we weren't laughing. When I was in the hospital, it rocked him because he could not understand why I would want to do what I did. When I was released, he and his wife were willing to book me a flight to anywhere I wanted to go so that I could heal. He was an excellent friend to me, but I was not a good friend to him. It ripped him apart when I decided to leave and never talk to him again. It wasn't until I decided to get help that I realized what I had done in our friendship. It was tough to process.

During this process, I realized that I had a lot to do with

the reasons I felt unloved. Mentally, I did not have the capacity to love anyone because I struggled to love myself. Since my childhood was so broken, I constantly tried to earn love and friendship, so none of the relationships had any substance. It had always been easy for me to walk away from any relationship with no regrets because I had never given my all to anyone or let anyone close to me. All of my relationships with my childhood friends and family had the same expectations. We knew the relationships would not last, and if they ended, I moved on to the next one.

I went my whole life not experiencing real relationships with guys who really cared about me. When it came to friendships with other men, I never trusted anyone because everyone I had ever trusted turned their backs on me in one way or another. I've had people who said they were friends to me lie on the legal documents that could have cost me my life, and friends who betrayed me by messing around with my girlfriends during my younger years. Though these seem to be small issues, both situations involved things I valued. One, you never tell on your friends, and two, you never mess around with your friend's girl. Although I struggled with other trust issues, I believed those situations kept me from fully trusting anyone. It took me years to see that growing up in the inner-city affected my view of relationships with friends.

Nelson and Martin were both good men, and they both

deserved to be valued in our friendship. If I could not value these two men in my life, you can only imagine how I treated everyone else. I never allowed myself to trust anyone, and I questioned every motive of everyone in my life. I spent many years in isolation, and though I hated people, I needed them for my temporary gain to fuel my success.

The only time I would feel important or loved was when I was on a stage speaking. I had the ability to captivate an audience, grabbing people's attention. I never felt I would have the opportunity to be free from the pain, but I desperately wanted others to experience freedom. I did not want them to go through life suffering the way that I did. At that moment, I did not understand how much damage I was causing. The people did not want to see me tell them about living free. They wanted me to actually live the freedom I talked about. I knew that was something I could not do in that season of my life. What I needed to do was walk away from it all and work on my own freedom first, which had been what this latest season of my life has been about.

During my freshman year of college, I met this amazing young lady. She was the best thing that ever happened to me at that time. I was a man from the hood, and she was a strawberry-blonde girl from the suburbs. She was everything I wanted in a woman and was so supportive. She believed in me and believed my past did not have to be my future. She could feel my brokenness and allowed me to be weak, finding ways to lift me up in tough times. She would spend hours in the library helping me with homework and pushed me to do better in school. I had come from a broken home and did not have a good relationship with my parents, but her family was amazing. Her mother would call me from time to time to check on me, and they treated me as if I was their own son. This was the first time in my life that I had ever allowed myself to attempt to experience love. The closer we got, the more afraid I became.

I always thought she was too good for me, and I did not want to cause her any harm. If she found out how hard I really struggled, she would leave. But looking back, I now know she would have done anything she could to make sure I was good.

One day I woke up and felt as though I needed to end the relationship. I made the decision to leave based on the fear of being loved and treated right. The day she came to visit me at my dorm, I immediately started an argument with her. I could see the hurt on her face, and when she got up to leave, I followed her to the door. I remember thinking if I put my finger in her face, she would leave me for good. I pointed my finger in her face and said some words I should not have said. That was the day our relationship ended, and rightfully so. I did not understand it then, but after I got healthy, I thought it was good that she refused to deal with my toxicity and knew her worth.

I grew up only seeing toxic relationships, and that's what I'd come to expect in my life. I did not believe I deserved to be in a healthy relationship—why would I when I did not see that modeled throughout my life. I would pursue relationships because of the excitement, but I lacked the energy to make the relationship work. If the other person did anything to hurt me, which is common in any relationship, I would shut down. In one particular relationship, I'd had a conversation with the other person about how I thought spitting in someone's face was the lowest and dirtiest thing you could do to someone. A few weeks later, during an argument, she decided to spit in my face. Though I stayed, our relationship was over that day. In another relationship, I was asked to pack my stuff and get out of the house after an argument. Due to my childhood, though I stayed, my relationship was over that day as well. I do not believe both of those situations deserved to be end-all situations, yet they were for me because I was unhealthy.

I spent most of my life in survival mode. I never lived because I was just trying to make it minute-to-minute, let alone day-to-day, from my younger years, all the way to adulthood. The truth was, I did not know how to live. I believe that is why it was easy to go through my life without healthy friendships and relationships. I functioned better in the toxic relationships, even though they were draining me in every aspect of my life. Ironically, I found it easier to walk away from healthy relationships than I did from the relationships that were unhealthy. Even knowing that, in the long run, the unhealthiness would have more of a negative impact on my life.

CHAPTER SIX

THERAPY

I was tired of riding the roller coaster of life. I was tired of being inconsistent while going through the highs and lows of life. I needed help. I had gone to therapy several times in my life, and I just could not connect with the therapist. Part of it had to do with me and the lack of trust I had in people. The other part had more to do with being a black man and not believing that therapy would work for me. So often, growing up, I would hear that black men are too strong for therapy and that no matter what life threw at us, we should be able to just get over it. I also had in the back of my mind the time I'd spoken to my guidance counselor and got the worse beating of my life. So I strongly believed therapy would not work for me because I could not open up and deal with the issues the real way.

When I thought hard about the "black men don't need therapy" belief, I realized that I had tried that approach to my life several times before, and it hadn't worked out that well because I was still suffering. I concluded that we needed therapy more than we wanted to admit because playing that tough-man role had led many of us down a dark path. Many men I'd seen growing up ended up in prison addicted to drugs, womanizers, or dead-beat fathers. Not because they wanted to but because they were only repeating the cycle of what we'd experienced. I did not want to continue that cycle; I wanted to be the one who broke it to help lead many of my brothers to a life of change and, ultimately, freedom.

After traveling and seeing many different parts of the world, I realized that it was not just black men who had problems with therapy, but it was men in general. I knew many people from many different races struggle through life. Many of my white counterparts had issues as well, though they may not have turned to the streets and gun violence as a result. Why would they, though, as that was not the pattern of life they had grown up seeing. However, many of them would turn to drugs and drinking, and often the womanizer complex. Why? Because that was the example their parents had set for them. When dad was mad at mom, he would just work or drink himself to death. We are all a product of our environment, regardless of where we come from.

Many men don't pursue the counseling side of things because they don't want another man to see that they are at a low point in their life. They may also have difficulty talking to their female counterparts because they don't believe women can understand what men go through. I know there were times in my life that I felt that way, and many of the men I ran into explained the same thing to me. We would rather keep everything in and not deal with it. And we are not going to talk to our women about it for fear of being reminded about it down the road. So, we continue to walk through life broken and messed up, faking like we got it all together.

I was tired of faking it and finally wanted to deal with my issues. I wanted to be the best father that I could be. I remember that day on November 2, 2015, when I became the father of two beautiful twin girls. I was so excited all the way up until they were born. When I held my girls for the first time, I was scared, my thoughts turning to my childhood and how I grew up. I did not want them to go through what I had gone through. Would I abandon them? Would I hurt them like my parents hurt me? I was happy to have them, but I was terrified of hurting them. When the nurse came to take them away from me, I followed because I did not want to be without them. Man, it was love at first sight. I knew I had to do the right thing. I needed to make sure that I was good.

A few days after they were born, I contacted a therapist and asked if I could schedule an appointment. Though I knew I had many people looking up to me and pushing me to follow my dreams, there was something about having my girls that made what everyone had been saying for years more tangible. When I walked into my therapy session, I was ready to unload—guns blazing. I shared with her everything about my life from childhood up until that day. I shared with her things that I had never shared with anyone a day in my life. From that day forward, we began to work on me.

I know you might want me to end the story right here and say it ended happily ever after. Not for me; realistically, it was tough. I wanted to give up, especially when we got to the first hurtful truth. She asked if I had ever been diagnosed with a mental illness. My first thought was, why does that matter? I just wanted help to get over everything; I wanted the quick fix. I told her of when I'd gone to the hospital the first time and was diagnosed with Bipolar Disorder and prescribed medication that made me hallucinate, which put me back into the hospital. I was finally taken off that drug, then I was told I did not have bipolar, but I suffered from Post-Traumatic Stress Disorder (PTSD), but I never followed up with it. I just tried to medicate myself with success and status. She decided to do her own research and came up with a more accurate diagnosis. She did not waste my time or hers. She said, "Well, I want you to know that you do have a mental illness. You have what we call C-PTSD (Complex Post-Traumatic Stress Disorder), which is similar to PTSD, but is when you face several traumatic situations over short or long periods of time." I immediately shut down and did not want to continue with the therapy. I did not go back for several months, even though I knew she was right. I just did not want to believe it yet.

When it came to being diagnosed with a mental illness, I never wanted to acknowledge that I was suffering. I had always felt as though I was stronger than I really was, and my pride would not let me feel weak. I never felt strong because I ignored my issues. Then I thought about all the stereotypes that came with having a mental illness. I watched how so many people in the field made fun of their patients and talked about the people on medication. I did not want that stigmatied to my name. I did not want to use my mental illness to excuse why I did what I did. Yes, there are reasons why people do and act the way they do. My symptoms were not an excuse but provided more context to why I thought and believed the way that I did. It was a clear understanding of my behaviors.

I decided to do my own research on C-PTSD and what some of the symptoms were. As I began to read, I was still in denial because I did not want to admit my situation's reality. The first thing I read was that a person with C-PTSD relives the trauma through flashbacks and nightmares. They avoid situations that remind them of the trauma, lose trust in themselves or others, and difficulty sleeping or concentrating. After reading that, I immediately realized that I was, in fact, the perfect candidate for C-PTSD. I'm talking in a major way. This was the explanation of my entire life and many of the symptoms I'd to endure in my life.

After researching, I accepted that I did have a mental illness and could not have the life I wanted if I didn't put in the work. So, I called and scheduled another appointment with my therapist. On the day of my appointment, I decided to admit that she was right and that I did have a mental illness and that I was a perfect candidate for it. To my surprise, she agreed. The next thing she said made me upset. She said, "I recommend you get on some medication. I am not saying that you will need it for the rest of your life, but you need it right now." I was so reluctant, but I knew I needed it. She reassured me that everyone did not have to know and I could go through life living normally. She believed that the medication would also help with the therapy process because of some of the topics we would have to discuss.

That week, I scheduled an appointment with my doctor and explained to her what my therapist recommended. I was given the prescription for my medication, and that was, by far, the longest and hardest walk to the pharmacy. When I handed the pharmacy tech my prescription, I was embarrassed and ashamed. She acted as if everything was normal, and I'd handed her a normal piece of paper. I was confused while I waited for my medication but brushed it off and went home. The next morning I woke up and started my medication, and I was so hurt. I remember thinking that I now had to take medicine because of what someone else did to me. I was just a kid and they were adults. I didn't understand why. This was not my fault.

In the next session, we discussed how I felt, and I shared with her that I was not feeling any different. I told her I was upset that I had to take a pill because of what other people did to me. I explained that it was not fair. She helped me see things from a different perspective. She told me to look at how much of my life I'd lost because I'd never gotten over what happened. Taking my medication would actually mean I was winning because I was now correcting and dealing with my life's pain and hurts. She then said we should increase my dose, and I followed her advice and upped my dosage.

After taking my medication for a few months, I noticed a huge difference in my life. I realized that I did not feel as on edge all the time. I noticed the flashbacks slowly happening less and less. I was more upbeat and relaxed, and I noticed that I wanted to be around people outside of brief conversations and my work environment. The medication was actually helping me. I felt as though I was living, which became more apparent when I asked myself if this is what normal people live like? The pill was no miracle worker, but it helped me to heal and get healthier.

I continued to go to therapy, and we continued to work

on many issues in my life. My life was not without its challenges. I had many issues arise through the process but what was apparent was that therapy was working, and I was changing and my life for the better. I began to find my worth and value myself the right way. And process the pain in my life. I realized that I'd suffered from mental illness ever since my first traumatic experienced. I did not know what life would be like without C-PTSD because I suffered daily from the symptoms. Though I'd had glimpses of success, my life felt horrible, but I was learning how to enjoy life and be ok with who I was and my struggles. I committed to staying in therapy, even if I felt I didn't need it and things were good. It was and has been great to actually heal the right way.

I don't want you to get the idea that therapy or medication was the miracle worker in itself. I had to put in work. If you aren't willing to work with it, it won't work for you. I had to realize how much of my life I'd lost and how many times I'd failed in my life. I knew it was time for me to experience life to its fullest. I knew that if I wanted to be a father to Jada and Jaylin, I would have to deal with my own past first. If I chose not to, I ran the risk of repeating the same cycle that my parents did to me.

While in therapy, I discovered there were some unhealthy relationships in my life at the time. I knew they needed to end, but just like I'd been my entire life, I was afraid to walk away.

But the more I sought therapy and healing, I knew what I needed to do. I asked my therapist what she thought I should do? She said, "Part of your healing is being able to make decisions for your life." I had a choice to remain unhealthy or pursue a healthy lifestyle. When I was able to make decisions that benefited my health and well-being, I knew that healing was taking place.

My approach to therapy was meant to be more like the relationship between a coach and a player. It is the coach's job to set the schedule for practices and its player's job to show up. It's the coach's job to teach the plays, but it's up to the player to execute the plays when it's game time. But when I walked into the therapist's office, I often wanted them to fix me and do all the work. When I realized that it was not their hurt, pain, or mental illness but mine, I was able to begin the healing journey, and I had someone to hold me accountable in the process.

When I hear people say therapy does not work, I often follow up with, "Did you work your therapy?" And like many people, I get this blank stare, like *what*? I usually follow up with, "Exactly, he or she does their work when you are in the office, but it's up to you to do the work when you leave. The reality is that not every therapist is going to work for you, but that does not me that no therapist will work." Sometimes it takes a while; it took me years to find someone that I connected with and trusted. But what I can tell you is that when you find the person you connect with, and you are ready for real change, your life will show it, as long as you are real, open, and honest in the therapy room.

There is nothing wrong with therapy. We all may need it at some point in our lives. Don't allow pride to stop you from going to see someone who has the expertise to help you find peace of mind and overcome your trauma. No one has to know what's shared in that room but you and the therapist unless you choose to talk about it. And for the men in the world, remember you are more of a man for going to therapy; you are harder and tougher than the men who refuse to go. What's hard about not confronting issues in your life is it actually makes you weak, and you become like every other man who succumbs to this stereotype of being soft and broken for the rest of your life and full of excuses. If it's one thing I have found to be true, it is that therapy is for the strong at heart. You did not get hurt alone, and you won't heal alone.

CHAPTER SEVEN

FORGIVING MY MOTHER

One topic that never came up in my therapy sessions was the topic of forgiveness. I was unwilling to discuss that issue, and since I never brought it up, we never talked about it. I don't know if it is the role of the therapist to approach that topic. It's something that one would have to wrestle with internally. But for me, it is a topic that is necessary for a person to be fully free from their offender or the person who caused them physical or emotional damage. Forgiveness is a part of our freedom process. Forgiveness is a must, not for our offenders, perpetrator, or family members' sakes, but for our sake. So that way, we can walk through life not being controlled by their actions towards us. It's a powerful sense of freedom and overcoming when we free ourselves from their actions.

I was doing an internship in a small country town called Live Oak, Florida, and I lived with a host family named the Durhams. This family was so awesome and really taught me a lot about healthy family dynamics. One day while I was outside weed eating, I went to Mr. Durham because I got this urge to have a conversation with my mom about forgiveness. Mind you, this is the first time I had ever in my life felt this way. With no hesitation, he gave me the keys to the car, and said go, who am I to stop you from making things right with your mother? So, I got in the car, and I drove an hour and a half to have a conversation. I wish I could tell you I was happy, but I wasn't. I was actually scared and afraid. Before this day, I hadn't talked to my mother for almost a year, and our last conversation did not go well. I had come home from school to visit, and she was sitting on the porch of my uncle's house. When I walked up on the porch, her face lit up with a smile.

"Oh, my son, came home to see me."

I ignored her and gave dap to everyone that was outside but her. She said, "Come give me a hug. I'm still your mother." If she wanted to be my mom, she would not be drunk and high right then. I looked at her and told her that she was my *birth mother*, but I'd had many moms in my life. When I said those words, I could see the hurt and pain on her face. I walked away that day feeling like what I did was right. I showed her, and I did not feel bad about it one bit. In my mind, if she wanted to be my mom, she would not have been under the influence.

As I was driving home that day, I continued to think about our interaction and how it probably affected her as I reflected on how the pain from our relationship had impacted me. Though I was succeeding in the world's eye, I knew that I could not move forward because of my relationship with my mother. I mean, I did have a right to feel how I felt, as I believed that most of my trauma came from her and her addictions. So, I felt she should apologize and ask *my* forgiveness.

When I arrived, my mother was home at the same house we grew up in. As I walked up, I could tell that she'd just finished getting high, and I could smell alcohol on her breath. I did not greet her like I did the last time I was home. I walked up to her and gave her a hug, and said, "Hey, Ma, I love you. How you doing?" and kissed her on her cheek. Her face lit up; she was so happy. I asked if we could talk, and she agreed.

I said, "Mom, I just want you to know that I forgive you for everything that you have done to me and every situation that I felt you put me in. I just want you to know that I don't want to carry this weight anymore, but I also don't want you to go through life feeling the same way. I forgive you. That night with your boyfriend really messed me up and all the other stuff. Like being homeless and watching you do drugs affected me also, but I can't keep blaming you for all the negativity in my life. I love you, and I want to start fresh from today with our relationship." We hugged and cried together for about 20 minutes. I gave her another hug, told her I loved her, and drove back to my host family's house.

That would probably be one of the longest drives of my life. I'd just forgiven my mom; I'd just forgiven the person who hurt me the most. I cried almost the entire ride back home. But I also felt as if someone took a brick off of my chest. From that day on, I would call and talk to her a few times a week. We would have actual conversations, and not the regular *how you doing*. Every time we got off the phone, we told each other, *I love you*. That may seem normal for some people, but before that day of our forgiveness conversation, I could remember on one hand the number of times my mother had told me she loved me. Now it felt real and genuine, my walls were down, and my heart was not filled with hatred. I always said, "I know your sickness is getting worse, but you have to hold on until I graduate college. I want you to see me walk across that stage." She would always reply, "Ok, baby, I'm going to try," but deep down, she and I both were doubtful as her health deteriorated.

Our doubts would prove true the following summer. I was working at a summer camp at my college and was having a blast until my family called the school and said I needed to come home because my mother was not doing well. After talking to my family, I found out my mother was very sick. I did not have a car at the time, but I knew I needed to get home. The bus was not running until the following day, and I did not know if it would arrive too late. So, one of my college friends, Sed, grabbed his keys and, with no hesitation, drove me 3 1/2 hours. I will forever be grateful to him for doing that for me.

We arrived at the hospital, and when I looked at my mother, I knew she was very ill. At that moment, I had so many emotions. Now that we were good and had a close relationship, she was going to die. But I could not think about myself; I had to focus on her. She looked at me and smiled because she was glad to see me. Though we did not have the best life together, I would serve her, and she would die knowing her son had truly forgiven her and loved her. She would die with dignity. The past did not matter at that moment.

Though it was painful watching her slowly fade in front of me, it would be some of the most memorable moments ever. We talked about everything, laughed so much, cried a bunch, and loved each other a lot more. She had ups and downs with her health. During this process, she temporarily lost her hearing and her sight. But she always knew when I was in the room. She could smell my cologne and would feel my arm.

"Who is this? This my son! Thank you for taking care of me." I would always tell her it was ok, and I felt honored to be there with her. I fed her, cleaned her, and made her bed for her. I would put her in her wheelchair and take her outside for some sun and conversation. I learned what the beauty of forgiveness was during this process. I also experienced grace as her hearing and sight returned after a few weeks.

After a month and a half, she took a turn for the worse. I came to the nursing home, and the doctors asked if they could meet with me. They told me my mom was not doing well, and she was in her final stages before death. I broke down, asking if there was anything more they could do, and was told no. They asked if I wanted her resuscitated if she passed while I wasn't there, and I declined. I left the doctor's office and walked to my mother's room.

She looked at me with a smile on her face and said, "Son, I know, you know I'm not doing well, but I am going to keep fighting. You are going to make it—you gotta make it for me. Don't let me down."

"Ok, mom, I will," and we hugged and talked as long as we could because she was in terrible shape.

The next morning, I wrote a letter to her because she was really struggling and fighting hard. In the letter, I told my mom it was ok to go now. I would be ok, and I knew she was tired. I ended the letter tell her I loved her. She read the letter and turned away from me. I walked outside to have some time to myself because I did not want her to see me break down and cried. I walked back into the room, and my mother looked at me, turned her head, and breathed her last breath. Though I was hurting, and I did not want her to go, I was thankful that I could love her through the process. By forgiving her, I was able to free myself and free her from some of the pain she'd felt for her mistakes as a mother.

I remembered a conversation with my mother where she revealed that she'd been molested as a young girl. She said the adults around her knew about it and did nothing to help. She admitted that she stayed in abusive relationships because she wanted to feel loved, even if it was painful. It was never apparent to her to love and protect us as she was never loved and protected herself. She used drugs to suppress her pain to not think about her mistakes and her sickness. I asked her why she never came to any of my games as a kid, and she'd revealed that she was embarrassed because of her sickness and drug addiction. After hearing her story, it made me have even more compassion for her. She was just repeating the cycle. Her funeral was the following Saturday, and I planned on leaving to go back to college right after the service. During the week of her funeral, I shared with my grandmother some of the things that my mother and I went through during my childhood. She told me that I sure had a story to tell. I did not know she would later confront one of the people that I had told her about. As I left my neighborhood to head back to college, I saw this white vehicle speeding, trying to catch up with us. The driver was yelling and waving for us to stop. So my friends pulled the car over. When I looked up, it was my mother's ex-boyfriend.

We both got out of the car at the same time, and he said,

"Man, your granny talked to me about all that stuff that happened when you was little." My first thought was, *this is my opportunity to get justice for what he did to me.* But he looked at me and said, "Man, I'm sorry for what I did to you and your mom that night. I did not think you would remember all that." I thought, *how do you think I was supposed to unsee and forget that night?* As I stood in front of him, it felt like I was still that same little boy from years ago. Though I had every right to be mad, I knew this was a huge moment for me. It was a test to see if I wanted the freedom I'd been longing for or did I want to remain that broken little boy. I'd suffered many years, and to hear my mother's boyfriend say to me that he never knew I remembered those things happening was mind-blowing. I thought to myself, *so I have been hurting and angry all these years for you to live your life like nothing ever happen. You have taken a lot of years from me, and you will not take anymore.*

This time, the ball was in my court and not in his hand. That day I realized I wanted freedom over revenge. I knew this moment was less about my feelings because I would have time to process those. This was more about healing and overcoming my demons. I replied, "I forgive you for what you did that night, man. But I remember everything, and it has affected my whole life, but thank you for apologizing." He apologized again, and we hugged. I whispered in his ear, "I forgive you now, forgive yourself." At that moment, the one man who was once a giant in my life broke down and was met with forgiveness instead of the bullets I'd once wanted to fire into him.

CHAPTER EIGHT

FORGIVING THEM

I had forgiven my mother and her boyfriend, but I still had one more chapter of forgiveness I needed to go through. I needed to forgive my father. I was not ready to forgive him during that time. It would actually take me years before I could gather the courage to do so. It did not happen the way I thought it would happen. I did not drive hours because I did not feel compelled to start the conversation. It was my 3-year-old daughters who opened my eyes and heart to forgive him. We arrived in Florida for my niece's graduation, and we were going to be there for several days. The girls started repeating, "Florida granddaddy! Daddy, we want to see granddaddy," so I called him, and we scheduled a day to go see him.

That day was a very powerful day in my life. As soon as my daughters saw him, they yelled, "Grandaddy! Grandaddy! Out—out daddy, we want granddaddy."

His face lit up as he said, "Come here, grandaddy's babies." The girls ran to him and embraced him with love.

They did not ask him if he'd been drinking that day. They didn't question his love or his motives. I had all those questions, but my daughters did not have to feel unsafe or threatened by him because they trusted me enough to protect them. And their conversations on FaceTime and over the phone were always filled with love and excitement. They remembered the pictures I showed them of him taking them to feed the cows bread, hugging and playing with them. It was the purest version I had ever seen of my father. But then I had a dark moment and thought if they only knew how he did not love me like that as a kid. Then I thought, why should they know him as I knew him? Maybe I should try to know him as they know him. As I looked at them, I wondered if it even mattered anymore? I needed to learn to love him with the same love that my girls did. I didn't need answers or excuses for what he'd done or hadn't done for me. I just needed to forgive him and love him from that day forward with pure love and no expectations of what I wanted in a father.

Though it may sound easy, it was a very tough choice to make. Deep down inside, I wanted answers. The first conversation we had to begin the restoration process was about him trying to kill my mother. The only thing he could say to me was to ask who'd told me that and that they were never supposed to tell. He was not willing to acknowledge his actions. I then asked why he'd always had to lie and why would he call if he was not going to show up? I explained to him how that made me feel like I was not important or wanted. He put his head down and could not respond. I realized that he was too hurt and angry to have a conversation like that. And honestly, I didn't need to have a conversation with him about the past. I knew it would not be beneficial for either of us, and I could forgive him and work on our relationship from that moment on with clear expectations and boundaries. Though I would never be able to get those moments back with him, I knew I didn't want those moments to affect how I parented my daughters. We still talk sometimes, and though he has not stopped drinking, I still love him as my dad.

To move forward in becoming the man I needed to be, forgiving my father was one of the biggest hurdles I had to jump. As a young black male who was rebellious against any authority, rules, regulations, and systems, I was bound to go through life the hard way, and battling mentally only increased those odds. Because of my father, I hated myself. I hated being black, I hated black men, I hated black authority. I wanted nothing to do with anything that reminded me of my father or my mother's boyfriend, who was also a black man. I developed a mindset that anything black was wrong. As hard as it was for me to admit, I turned my back on the culture, and my brothers became my enemies. It was easier for me to hurt those who looked like me because I had been hurt by those who looked like me.

After being released from the hospital in 2009, I arrived back to my old neighborhood with a suitcase, no place to live, and twenty dollars in my pocket. I was so embarrassed because I felt that the people who once looked up to me for making it out were looking down on me. It was the most humbling experience I'd had in a long time. I walked through my neighborhood and stated, I guess it's true; we all do come back eventually. I realized that I was no different from drug dealers, drug addicts, prostitutes, and alcoholics. We were all just scarred-up people dreaming that one day we'd have peace of mind from the trauma of our childhoods.

If there's one thing I knew how to do, it was to hustle. I picked up the phone, and I called one of my friends I used to sell drugs with. I said, "Hey man, I need you to come through and talk with me." About half an hour later, he pulled up to my neighborhood. When I got in the car, I told him that I needed to get back in the game for a little bit, at least until I could get back on my feet.

He looked me in my eyes and said, "Naw, man, I can't do that." He reached in his pocket and gave me some cash and said, "I don't know what you're going through, but I want you to know we look up to you. We talk about you all the time, so I'm going to need you to get your mind right and follow your calling, bro." I was embarrassed and put my head down. He said, "And I'm going to need you to keep your head up. We need you."

I did not have a car at the time, so I walked to Pops' house. Pops was a man who called me his hero for making it out of the neighborhood and going to college. I walked into his room and began to cry because I felt so lost and afraid of the mental state I was in. His first words to me were, "Oh, one of my heroes came to see me."

"Look at me," I said. "I'm not a hero no more. I don't have anything, and I'm mentally struggling. I just tried to start selling drugs again."

He replied, "You have gone through worse; why give up now?"

I said, "I don't know if I have it in me anymore." "So, what are you going to do?"

I looked at him with anger in my eyes and said, "I hate my own people. For years I have not felt comfortable in my skin as a black man. I judge my father, uncles, and family members, but I am no different. I am a successful mental case." That day, I realized not only did I need to forgive my father, but I needed to ask for forgiveness for all the young black men I'd failed along this journey. Knowing I'd had the opportunity to help them, but instead judged them. I learned one of the darkest mental issues in my life was hate, and if I wanted to move forward, I had to forgive and heal.

When I was able to heal from my father's hurt, my eyes opened to my struggles with self-hatred. Once I stopped blaming him for everything he'd done wrong in my life and acknowledged my issues, the truth about my struggles became real. I was able to see how my self-hatred elevated my mental deterioration.

The last thing I had to do was forgive the women who had molested me. I knew a conversation with them would not be granted and would not go over well. But I still needed to forgive them. My therapist recommended that I write them a letter and burn it. I wrote letters as if I was talking to them face to face and explained that I no longer wanted to carry this pain nor allow it to hinder any other relationships I had in the future. I forgave them and no longer wanted to give them control over my life. I ripped the letter up, and I threw it in the trash, knowing that would be the last time I had to have that talk.

Forgiveness is a scary subject, and many people get very emotional when the topic comes up. One day, I was speaking at a summer camp, and a young lady came up to me and said, "I heard you talk about forgiveness. Does that me I have to forgive my stepfather who molested me from the ages of 6 to 12?" with hesitation, she looked at me and said, "I don't think I can do that.

"Look at all he has taken from your life. Do you want

him to continue to take away from your life?" I asked.

"No," she replied.

"Forgiveness is not about him, but it's about you freeing yourself from the pain that he has caused you. He will always have control over you until you forgive. In order to heal from what he has done, forgiveness is a must." She broke down at the table that day, and we walked through what forgiveness looks like.

Forgiveness is not about the other person as much as it's about you releasing the control of what they have done to you. When you walk around bitter and ashamed for what you had to go through, the person who did those things still has control over you.

When you forgive someone, that does not mean you need to build a relationship with them. In many cases, the only time forgiveness results in a relationship afterward is in close relative relationships, and only if sexual abuse was not present. Let's free you from thinking that you have to build new relationships with your perpetrator. NO! This is a time when you can be selfish with your forgiveness and whatever it takes to free yourself. However, if there are relationships that can be restored, relationships that make forgiveness that much more powerful, give it a try. When you forgive, remember to set clear boundaries in the relationship to promote a healthier lifestyle.

CHAPTER NINE

FORGIVING MYSELF

I find it ironic when we try to understand to what extent our actions have affected the other person. That is something we will never be able to measure because every wound affects the individual differently. When we say to ourselves that it was not that serious, how do we really know how bad it was when we are not the person we hurt? That helped me realize that I could not waste time thinking about how it affected the other person but helped me focus on what I did to hurt them.

This would make my journey of forgiving myself easier to obtain.

When we think about forgiveness, we often think about how we have to forgive others for what they have done to us. We rarely think about how our actions have affected people. Shame and regrets we carry for our mistakes in our own lives. Another component of forgiveness is us being able to forgive ourselves. And for many years, that was hard for me to do. I felt that I was justified to act and live how I did because of what I had gone through. I was following the trend of our world today, hurt people hurt people. I was hurting people and knew what the effects could be and how they ran the risk of being damaged like me. I'd witnessed it time and time again in conversations with others as they shared their personal experiences. What I thought to be uncommon; therapy and conversations helped me see how common hurting people becomes a vicious cycle.

I sent a friend request to a young lady I went to elementary school with via Facebook. She excepted the request, and I sent her a message asking how she was doing. We started the conversation with small talk, discussing our lives with kids and life as adults. But later in our conversation, she stated to me that I was very mean in school. And that because of me, there were days that she did not want to come to school. I knew that was not the only consequence of my decisions, as she went on to say that she was lucky that she was able to overcome me being a bully and mean to her.

Most adults would have made excuses as it being normal childhood behavior, but whether or not they believed it to be normal, it did affect people in a negative way. My first response was to immediately tell her that I was going through a rough time in my life, and I was taking it out on her. I knew that would not do any justice for what she'd felt or had gone through. I apologized to her for my actions and how they had affected her life, and I took full responsibility. She stated she was very thankful for my apology, and though it did not cure everything, it was the beginning of healing for her.

Then I remembered a young man I went to the same school with, who my friends and some family members would pick on daily. I had come into town to speak at my grade school and ran into his mother. I asked her how he was doing, and she looked at me with this overwhelming hurt in her eyes. She explained that he was in prison and that he was addicted to drugs before going to prison. I knew some of his life choices were because of the actions of my friends and me. I wasn't ready to have that conversation with her at that time, though. She looked at me and said she was proud of the man I was becoming, and I had come a long way. She was right about many of the changes I'd made. What we both silently acknowledged at that moment was how my old behaviors had affected the life of her son.

I remembered fighting with him and developing a hatred for him, even though he'd done nothing to deserve the treatment. We would argue and fight all the time, and most of the fights were because of me. His family tried everything they could to get the behavior to stop. They tried mediation, they called the police and got them involved, but nothing would work. To this day, I don't know why I hated him so much, other than I needed someone to push the pain on.

One day he got tired of it, pulled a knife on me, and put it to my neck. If he had killed me that day, I don't believe he should have done any jail time, just based on how I treated him growing up. He was not like that, so he dropped the knife and ran. I went to his house and knocked on the door in an attempt to get to him. His sister answered the door, screamed in fear, and closed it. I had not just affected him, but his family as well. My treatment of him caused a ripple effect with the people who raised and grew up with him. I spent many nights knowing what I did to that family was wrong.

I felt guilty that I was given a second chance at life, while the two people I talked about above would only be two of the hundreds of people I hurt throughout my life. To be able to live a life in peace, I had to get to a place where I could forgive myself. If I didn't, then there was no way for me to have the opportunity to experience a new life. I couldn't change what I'd done in the past; I could only do what I could with the future ahead of me. If I lived with regret and shame, I would only cripple myself.

Does everyone deserve a second chance at life, then? Does everyone deserve to re-write their story? The answer to that question is yes! The hardest part for many will be if others will allow them to forget about the mistakes they've made. Just because you forgive yourself does not mean the people you hurt will ever forgive you. And that is something you will not have any control over, but that does not mean you have to walk around holding onto your past based on how someone else deals with it.

I had a young man come to see me who'd taken the life of another person. He asked me if he would ever be free to live his life again? I looked at him and said, "Yes, but it is up to you. You have to find peace within because no matter how much you change, to many people, you will always be a murderer. However, that does not mean you have to live like one. You can be in prison for a long time and still live with more peace than the people on the outside." I watched that young man fight every day to try and be a different person, and though the world would remember his actions, he would still have the opportunity to live a life of peace. And yes, he deserves the opportunity to be free.

I had to get to a place where I could move forward, but it was as if my legs were shackled together: one shackle was the forgiving others, and the other was forgiving myself. I found it easier to forgive others, but the end of that cuff was weighed down by past mistakes and failures. Walking around with unwanted mental pressure is more than enough to break a person down. No matter what you have done in your life, we all deserve a second chance, though many people may disagree with me. I would just ask them if they had gone through their entire life without hurting anyone? The answer to that question would most likely be no.

When we don't deal with our past, the ones that come behind suffer from it. That would become a reality of how my not dealing with my past affected the future. My sister called me one morning and said that my little cousin had been shot. He depended on me to help him, and I often felt that I'd let him down. He went through several surgeries as they tried to save his life, but after about a month, he passed away from complications from getting shot. I was not expecting that phone call because he was not involved in any trouble. He worked two jobs and took care of his kids.

I took a trip to see him while he was in the hospital. When I walked into his room and saw him on the machine, my first response was to make the person who did this pay. Then I realized he may not have been in that bed if I would have had my life together and fulfilled my promise to him. After he graduated high school, we'd discussed that he would move in with me and attend college, and I would support him. I was financially able to uphold my part of the bargain during that time of my life. But before he graduated high school, I went through my own troubles and struggled with my health causing me to lose everything.

The day my sister called and told me he had passed away, my heart broke, and the feeling lasted a long while. I carried that pain for a few months, but thankfully I was on my healthy journey and in therapy at the time. Instead of taking several steps backward, I took even more steps forward. I made it my mission to help as many people as I could make it through life. As *payback* to the people who took you from me, I will do my best to help 10 million people find freedom. Instead of carrying guilt, I carry his memory with me every day, and it motivates me to continue to keep pushing. Though I wish the outcome would have been different, I couldn't change it, but I can change the future. I have made an effort to honor and value people and do the right thing, even when it hurts.

CHAPTER TEN

FEAR OF HEALING

One of the questions I get asked all the time is, why did it take me so long to heal? The quick answer is always I did not know *how* to heal. Though the statement is true, it is far more complex than that. I don't know how many people live with mental illness, screaming and begging for help as they continue to struggle. People are searching for answers to ways to pursue a healthy lifestyle and control their mental illness without it controlling them. But after years of forming bad habits that only added to their suffering, they, like me, are operating in fear, which makes healing look impossible. Not only did I form bad habits, but as you know, I was afraid to face the truth of having a mental illness. I thought the more success I achieved, the higher the chance the pain would go away. I was comfortable suffering because it had been happening my whole life, and I was afraid to start over. My trauma was my security blanket, and having peace of mind was something I never knew was possible.

I'd never seen anyone stand on a stage and yell, "I have a mental illness!" and say it with confidence and pride. Most of the time, when it's bought up, it's with a negative attached, like a school shooting, psychiatric hospitals, or someone committing suicide. Mental health is rarely normalized in social spaces. I knew I was not normal, and I knew I was suffering deeply, but I would rather have suffered in silence than to allow my name to be mentioned with such negativity behind it. I had an image to protect. How could someone claim to be a person of influence and struggle at the same time? I was afraid to heal because I wanted to protect my image. If people knew that I had C-PTSD, they would judge me and use it against me. I'd suffer this long, so I was not in a rush to get any better, and my facade had led me to many successes. I adopted the "fake it till you make it" attitude.

Most people who struggle with mental illness often find themselves addicted to drugs, drinking, or have sexual addictions. I did not struggle with any of those; my drug of choice was success. I felt that the more successful I became, the less my struggles mattered. You've never heard anyone come up to someone after a sports game and say, man, that was a good game, so what mental illness do you struggle with? Nor has anyone asked a person who was considered higher rank than them, what mental struggles do you have? When you see someone who has reached success, you want to know how they got where they're at. I needed the success to cover up my deepest, darkest wounds.

I've come to the belief that no matter how successful a person is, if they have a mental illness, it will always show itself. Why? Because anything unbalanced cannot sustain the façade of being balanced. Though I had reached the top in almost every company or organization I had ever worked for, I had also hit rock bottom each and every time. Though I have had some amazing relationships that started off well, they also ended. Though I was not the only component to all of these things ending, I and my mental illness played a role in their demise.

After doing some deep soul searching, I've now realized that many of those jobs could have lasted if I would have been honest with myself and my struggles. I had a phone conversation with my former pastor of the church, where I was the youth pastor. To this day, he has remained consistent in his love for me. He that it was hard to watch a young man so gifted and talented suffer the way that I did, and he would have been willing to walk through anything with me. Though I wanted to doubt those words, I knew deep down they were true because even in my darkest moments, he and his wife did a lot to try and walk through some of the dark times with me.

No matter how successful a person is, pain and mental illness will never fade, never just go away. It's no different than the people who are doing drugs; when the high is gone, the pain becomes a reality, and they're right back where they were before. I remember one speaking engagement I went to where I was invited to speak at a local middle school. I walked into the cafeteria and saw over 100 students. These were not your normal students. They were a part of a drop-out prevention program. I grabbed the mic and told them my story and how I had overcome and made it out of my neighborhood. That day was very impactful for all those students. I knew because a week later, I received cards and handwritten notes from all of the kids who were in attendance. I remember one of the letters from a young girl who stated that she was contemplating suicide the day I came to her school and that my story had given her hope, and now she had found a reason to live. She encouraged me to continue to share because I was helping a lot of people.

What that young girl will never know is that I was minutes away from attempting to end my life before reading her letter. She would never know that she had actually saved *my* life. That moment taught me about using success as my drug to escape from the pain because when you are at the top, you have a lot of influence, and people are looking up to you. If I had been successful in killing myself, I would have affected so many lives because I have had the opportunity to reach many people. The drug of success and reaching people while battling mental illness is a dangerous playground. Though I was afraid to heal because of the success, I was one suicide attempt away from causing more trauma and pain to those who looked up to me.

Another reason I was afraid to heal was that I had become comfortable in my pain. I had lived twenty-five years hurting, so the idea of being healthy was not appealing to me. I did not know what living a healthy lifestyle looked like. I had managed to live this long with mental illness, so what would changing to heal do for me now? It would mean me becoming a new person, and I did not know if I wanted that for my life. It's crazy how someone can battle with thoughts of choosing freedom over being stuck in their pain. But what many people don't know is that when a person becomes aware that they have struggles, they are more prone to take several steps backward before they are willing to take a single step forward. And I was that person who was afraid to take that step forward.

When I was twelve years old, I broke my ankle playing football. I was taken to the hospital, and after completing x-rays, they told me that I would need surgery to repair the broken bones. I woke up from surgery and looked under my blankets and started screaming really loud, "My leg, my leg! They took off my whole leg!" The nurse came over and asked me what was wrong, as she thought I was screaming from withdrawals from the medication. I said, "No, my leg! They took my leg off in surgery." She told me they had not removed my leg, and it was just a cast that had to be brought up to the middle of my thigh because I'd torn ligaments, and they needed to heal as well. This made no sense to me for a cast to be all the way up to my thigh, and it was just my ankle that was broken. I'd expected the cast to only come between my knee and calf.

I had to wear the cast for about six months until they removed it. The day they cut it off, my leg was full of dead skin and was about the same size as my arm. And it smelled, like really, really horrible. The doctor came in and said, "I reviewed the x-ray, and your leg has healed and will function like normal in a few months." I looked down at my leg and looked at the doctor, wondering if we were looking at the same leg. When I left the office, I left using my crutches, and a few weeks later, I was still using my crutches as if I had my cast on. Then I realized that if I kept using my crutches, my leg would never reach its full potential, and the process of healing would take longer. That also applied to my healing from my past. I could either use my past as a crutch or heal and live a good life. Like my broken leg healed, we can also heal from our trauma and live well with mental illness. Though there is a process to healing, taking months for some and years for others. But if we never get rid of the crutch called pain, we will never know what healing is supposed to look and feel like!

CHAPTER ELEVEN

THERE'S NOTHING YOU CAN'T OVERCOME

If there's one thing I am thankful for, it's that through my struggles with mental illness and battles with suicide, I did not succumb during my attempts. I am thankful that I found the courage to fight and not give up. That I pursued healing by forgiving those who hurt me, going through therapy, and choosing to take my medication every day that I woke up. I've also gotten over the pressures of caring what people thought of me, and I can live my purpose without wearing a mask.

When I reflected on my journey of getting to this point, I never thought that I would see and know the freedom that I have now.

I knew that I had arrived at a real place of freedom the day I woke up and looked at myself in the mirror and was able to say, *I Love Me*. I loved the healed me. I loved the free me. I loved the mental illness me. Why? Because at that moment, I no longer was the victim but the victor. I had reached a place of the overcomer. I was no longer bound by the trauma and turmoil of my life. Though I will forever carry some of the scars from my past, they are scars and not open wounds. The scars represent the healing and remind me of what I have overcome.

For many years I'd believed that it was impossible for me to live in peace and have mental freedom. The first step I made to overcome my past had been to be willing to admit I had an issue with mental illness. As a black male, I wrestled long and hard with that, but I knew I couldn't hide anymore. I knew there was no opportunity for me to overcome without acknowledging that first. I had tried to heal myself, tried to pray it away, tried to succeed it away, and nothing worked. The reality was it was not going anywhere, and no matter what I tried to do, it would always be a part of me. When I took the step to admit that I had faced my first challenge, I started overcoming it. Struggling with depression, PTSD, bipolar, or any other mental illness is not a bad thing. It becomes a bad thing when it's not diagnosed or goes untreated. They don't just go away either, but they do get better when we take the time to work on them and heal.

I was afraid of what people would think of me when they found out my greatest struggle. But when I stopped thinking about what people would think of me and focused on what I thought about myself, I was able to see the true value in my life. Just like me, many people in the world struggle with what people think of them. This is true for people who don't have mental illnesses, but it is worse for people who struggle mentally. I was more concerned about my self-image and people's opinion of me more than I was concerned about being whole. I realized that I was protecting something that wasn't real and hating people for loving what was not real. And the people who were supposed to be in my life would love me for me regardless of my mental struggles because they were more concerned about me as a person. This was a huge hurdle for me in healing and overcoming because it took so much unneeded pressure off me. I was able to take off my mask and be the real me.

The day it became apparent to me was when someone who claimed to love me hurt me in a way that attempted to damage me and some important people in my life. During this meeting, she looked at the people in the room and told them I was bipolar and suicidal—the moment she said that, I immediately became angry and upset. But then I realized she was wrong because, actually, I had C-PTSD, and I *was* suicidal, but it had been over 9 years since my last attempt. At that moment, I was not afraid to stand up for myself, be honest about my past struggles, and was also able to talk about how I'd overcome them. I got a letter from a professional that expressed how hard I had worked to overcome those struggles. That was the first moment in my life that I could see the fruit from me facing my issues.

One of the biggest lessons learned from that situation was that as you are overcoming and building your confidence, be mindful that some people will try to keep you in that dark place and dark moments of your life. Part of overcoming and being mentally healthy is not being afraid of letting go of the people who won't let you grow. When you are hurting and not stable, people around you know they have the upper hand to manipulate and control you. In those moments, when others are trying to use your struggles against you, the best defense is to be truthful. Look at them and say, "You're right about my past struggles, but you forgot to mention one thing. I am overcoming and controlling my mental health." I had to overcome every day until one day, I looked up and realized that I had finally made it.

My triumphs had nothing to do with what others thought about me. They were not there during the many nights I contemplated and attempted suicide. They were not there the nights I faced those traumatic experiences. My overcoming had everything to do with me being able to live a healthy. Me being able to live a life of freedom and have mental peace. I realized that I was giving people too much credit and too much room to dictate my life. Whether I dealt with my mental illness or not, everyone around me would go on and live their lives. I wanted them to, but my focus needed to be on being the best version of myself and not the version everyone else wanted me to be. Though I did not know what that looked like, I knew it had to be better than what I had always done.

As I grew and lost the idea of needing people and living a lie, I had to learn to be comfortable with the new me. Though life for me was getting better, I wrestled with going back to the old me because a healthy me was foreign. For many months, it was like playing tug-of-war. One minute, I found myself being strong and leading the way, but then other days, I found myself losing the war; my past was pulling on me hard. Telling me I was strong now and I did not need my medication, so I would believe it and stop taking them. And I found myself back down the same dark road, isolated from the world and trying to fight it alone. Like all the other times, I found myself losing again, and I would pull myself together and continue the fight.

One day while playing this game of tug-of-war, I looked at the end of the rope and stared my past straight in the face. I realized that I truly had the power to win this game. All I had to do was let go of the rope because I did not have to wrestle anymore if I did not want to. That day came when I finally allowed myself to feel and know what healthy living looked like. Some people feel as though when someone wrestles and fights with an issue, it has to be bad. When it comes to mental illness, I have learned that it's a good thing. Because in some of the wrestling, that person will see and feel some components of healthy living. I would rather wrestle than be in a comfortable place. Again, this is about someone on a journey to get whole.

For many people, being whole and having a healthy mind is normal and has been their entire life. For a person that has or is struggling with an untreated illness, being healthy is like a foreign language. It's almost as if they have not been able to walk for years and now have to learn to walk again. What our world deems normal is not so normal in our eyes. And when you are healing and learning what normal looks like as an adult, it's even more complicated because you still have bills, have a job, may have kids, spouses, or friends. Not only do we have to adjust, so do the others around us.

I realized that I had been married twice and never loved someone. Because I had never known what real love was. I never even loved myself, so how could I have loved someone else? In my relationships, all I did was model what I was told a relationship was all about. As a man in a relationship, you worked to provide, sometimes be intimate, opened the door for her, bought gifts, and sometimes went on dates. I'd forgotten all about the trust and friendship part, so when I told someone I loved them, I was in love with the things that I could do for them and not in love with the person. When I left a relationship, I was never really affected emotionally because I was never involved emotionally. My so-called love would shut off the very first time I was hurt or negatively affected by something they did or said. My pain and abuse radar would tell me to abort the mission. This was not only my relationships with the opposite sex but in my friendships as well.

Because I was so unhealthy, I had unhealthy relationships with people. I needed people to stroke my ego and make me feel as though I was normal. But I never allowed myself to be open to building genuine relationships. I gave everything to the people who never had my best interests at heart, but I would crush and hurt those who were genuine to me. I believed that all I needed in this life were three people: me, myself, and I. But part of the overcoming process was realizing that I needed people. I needed real relationships. That would mean I needed to open myself up and allow people to get to know me for me.

When I was unhealthy, I did not care who or when things I shared with people. As I improved, I realized that I did not need a million people on my team or beside me. I needed a few people who I could trust to walk and do life with. Facebook cuts you off at 5000 friends, and for me to remain healthy and overcome, I took the five and gave them back the three zeros. What I've learned on this journey was that I didn't need 5000 people to help me continue to heal and beat my mental illness. I needed a few people who knew my highs and lows and could walk with me through them. And the five people in my core needed to be pushing for better and striving to be healthy.

One of my biggest struggles with that was I had to let some people go, and some of those people would be offended. I could no longer worry about who was offended by me pursuing a life of healthy living. I had to think about my health and realize that not everyone who started with me would finish with me. That is not an easy part of the process, but it is a much-needed part. When I was overcoming, I couldn't worry about who I was offending, but I knew that once I became whole, they would understand.

If there's one thing I've had issues with my entire life, it was consistency. I was all over the place. I had a dream for every day; I woke up with a new daily mission. Nothing in my life was consistent. But I knew that for me to overcome, I had to remain consistent. The only way I would be able to succeed was to be committed. If you think it was hard for someone who was mentally stable to be consistent, think of how hard it was for someone like me. I talked a good game, but man, I had a hard time following through. Like many people, when I did not complete a task, I always had an excuse as to why I could not get things done. Though I felt I had a good excuse, I never told people what my real excuse was. Can you imagine? Someone could ask me why didn't I finish this project.? And my response would be, "Oh, because I've got childhood trauma and C-PTSD that I've never dealt with." Though I would have been telling the truth, no one was going to buy that.

When I realized how powerful consistency was when it came to overcoming, it was life-changing. I thought about how I constantly deal with issues and how damaging they were to my life. Just like inconsistency added more turmoil, consistency added health benefits and was instrumental to me experiencing freedom.

CHAPTER TWELVE

POWER OF HEALING

It's a powerful thing when a person who has suffered for so long finds a way to live their purpose, especially when they find their dream as a whole being and not as a broken one. I often think about all that I have accomplished being unhealthy, and it was a lot. While being mentally unstable, I would be the first person in my family to graduate high school in over twenty years. I was the first person ever to graduate college in my family; though it took me 6 years to finish, I accomplished my goal. I completed both of these goals with a learning disability, which I was able to overcome. Many people did not think I was capable of accomplishing those goals, but I did. Though I had many struggles to overcome, there was always a glimpse of hope that I would one day do so. The little accomplishments are what gave me hope to continue to push through in the toughest of times.

So, when I got the opportunity to speak on stage, it had a different meaning. Before, I needed people to give me the energy to get through it. I considered myself the Terrell Owens of speaking, and I was good at what I did but very inconsistent and lived a life controlled by the vibes. Every opportunity I get now, I don't look at what I can get from them or what energy they bring. I look at the reason they came, and many of them come to my events because they are suffering and struggling themselves and need to see that there is hope. Others come because they have family members and friends who struggle with mental illness and want to know how to help them. So when I look into the crowd, it's not about what they can give me but what I can give them. From my life experiences, struggles, pain, and failures, I hope that they won't make the same mistakes. I also encourage them by presenting a man who used to wake up every day wishing he was dead that now wakes up thankful for each morning he's alive.

Mental illness does not disqualify you from living your dream. What it does is determine how you will accomplish your dream and consistently live it out daily. There are many people with mental issues running businesses, leading companies, and playing professional sports. Some are doing it well, and others are running their companies into the ground. The difference between the two is who is in control, the person, or their mental illness. The dream that you have inside of you will not die or go away. It will remain within you regardless of where you are mentally. But for you to be successful, it is waiting on your surrender to help and commitment to the process of healing.

Wow! I wish I could put my life on a jumbo screen to allow you to physically see the difference overcoming my pain and trauma has made in my life. And to be honest, many people have the same story as me, if not worse, who did not make it through their trauma. A difference between me and the people who did not make it is that I decided to face my trauma head-on. And I made a choice to stop running from my pain but face it to gain healing so it would no longer hinder my dream, passions, and life. In the midst of all my struggles and failures, I found a way to overcome them. That is what winners do.

When I think about all of the young black boys who have the same story as me, just with different outcomes, it is hard for me to stay silent. I think about the darkness they've had to go through in their lives. I think about how they, too, had dreams and how their outcome would have been different if they would have had someone to coach them through the healing process. If they could have seen that they were people and not just broken black boys. I am that coach now, though.

Now that I have healed, my dream has become to use my journey and struggles to help others break free. I want people to know that they can dream and live a good life despite past trauma and mental illness. Though I have failed in the past, I am thankful for my failures for every struggle because I have gone from struggling mentally to having mental toughness. When I dreamt of being a speaker, I never thought it would have been in this capacity and with this topic. I have spent many of my years on this earth hurting people. I will now get the opportunity to watch the world heal one life at a time.

I often get asked if I regret the things I went through? If you had asked me that question a few years ago, I would have said yes. But after healing, I realized that everything I'd gone through was for a reason and would be used to bring peace to the lives of many people. And if people with mental illnesses begin to realize how normal they are regardless of their age, gender, or race, then I am living my dream every day. My goal is to start to see colleges care more about the athlete's well-being by acknowledging any mental illness and trauma more than their talents. That school would provide support and a real understanding of their students' background, focusing on trauma awareness. I hope the court system focuses on helping people not become a product of the system but to develop healthy living habits.

Most of all, I want people who battle with mental illness to know that they are not alone. That even though they may feel like they are the only ones in the world struggling, that is far from the truth.

I knew that I was born to be great. My life was not about

me because I was born to impact this earth. I needed to take the time to heal. There were people worldwide depending on me to tap into my gift and offer them the freedom that they sought their entire lives. That became very apparent to me one day in a focus group at work. I looked at a group of broken young men and told them, "I was just like you. I made some of the same mistakes you're making today. But I found it in myself to turn my life around and seek a better life for myself. I stopped making excuses and made moves because I believed I could be and do better."

The group was silent until one of the *tough* kids spoke, "We love it when you come to work because we know you are going to hold us accountable and give us that real talk. If we had someone like you in our lives on the outside many of us would not have ended up in here. We've never had a black man be as real with us as you have. Don't get stuck here; this ain't you. You can come back here and talk to us, but man, go live your dream. You taught us a lot whether we listen to it or not. Somebody out there will." And for the next ten minutes, several kids told me the same thing, agreeing with what he'd said. I was rocked by how much I'd impacted these kids, kids people had said would only be criminals for the rest of their lives. That day those *misfits* and *throw-away* kids spoke more life into me than I'd had in a long time. They confirmed my healing was showing.

I knew I was in a healthy place in my life, but I was more afraid of losing the healthy person I'd become because I was there. This was because I had never followed my dream from a healthy place. My C-PTSD symptoms would increase when I was pursuing a dream, and being in unhealthy relationships did not help either. I knew that I had to make some changes before putting effort into living my God-given purpose. Over a few years, I began to make those changes while maintaining my juvenile detention center job. Therapy was a must, and taking my medication was a no-brainer, so my journey into healthy living would become the norm. Though many people around me did not understand many of the changes that I was making to get healthy, I did not let that hold me back. I continued to press towards the goal.

Pain, trauma, and mental illness do not disqualify you from living a good life full of promise, happiness, and joy. From the day you were born, it was the life that was promised to you. But with a world full of hurting people, it would only be a matter of time before you felt pain, experienced that trauma, and/or battled mentally. When I decided to control my life and not lay down and quit, I became a stronger man that day. I decided that I was going to take all of my pain and turn it into my passion. Instead of being mentally weak, I was going to live a life of mental toughness. I wouldn't focus on how good it would have been to die and end it all. Instead, I was going to work through the tough times and live my life to the fullest. And for everyone that had let their struggles destroy their lives, I was going to live a life that showed people that you can take your life back from the people who'd hurt you and live up to your full potential. Though I had made many mistakes, failed miserably, and hurt some people along this journey of healing, I forgave the people who had hurt me, and I had forgiven myself for the pain that I caused others. I am going to live the rest of my days without any regret. It is a powerful thing when a person who has suffered so long finds a way to live their purpose. It is inspiring to find their dream as a person who has become whole versus being a broken individual. I am now that whole individual living my dream and purpose.

CHAPTER THIRTEEN

UNHAPPY DREAMER

When I began to heal, I thought everyone would be happy for the changes I was making. But one thing that became apparent was that not everyone would celebrate or be happy for my changes and growth. And those were people who benefited more from me when I was down and at my lowest point in life. So, for you to move forward, you must be comfortable losing them. It is better to lose people who are of no help to your growth than to lose yourself trying to please them. The healthiest version of you is more important than being unhealthy to make them happy. What you will find as you heal is that those people who try to keep you down are unhealthy themselves.

I remember the day someone who claimed to love and care for me looked me in my face and told me that their goal in life was to destroy me. After that day, I decided that I would fight hard to build a relationship with that person. Even though I knew the relationship was unhealthy and detrimental to my physical, spiritual, and mental health, I was willing to put my sanity on the line to make that friendship work. At the end of the day, the relationship contributed to me falling into a deep depression, triggering my C-PTSD. I had many people around me screaming and yelling in my ear to fight and make it work, but the whole time I was losing myself. I followed the advice of many and did not follow my heart's desire because I was afraid to fail. When I decided to think about my well-being and health, I lost a lot of people and faced a lot of judgment but regained myself.

As I grew after the above situation, I decided to find a few people that I could open up to, a select group of people. In the midst of me opening up and sharing some of my deepest struggles, I again found myself being betrayed and stabbed in the back. Everything that I had opened up about with a few people in the group became a weapon they used against me in the long run. Anytime tension or issues arose, they quickly reminded me of my past struggles and mental battles. If I had a rough moment or tough day, I would get asked if I was taking my medications. Life could not just be happening to me, nor could the day just be tough. They would also take those conversations to other people, spreading lies, rumors, and gossip. The unhealthy me would have tried to find a way to make the relationship work for fear of the backlash I would receive. The healthy me knew it was time to cut ties and protect everything I had worked hard to gain.

I decided to cut them off because I felt betrayed and the trust was broken. I walked around with a target on my back, and every chance they got to hit the bullseye, they did. I knew the relationship was unhealthy on so many levels, and I had no choice but to think about my well-being and healing process. Regardless of what they did or tried to do, my character, hard work, and dedication spoke louder than their gossip. Everyone has a past and has made mistakes. When I was unhealthy, I made a lot of mistakes. Now that I am healthy, I have learned to guard my progress and protect my peace in the midst of development and growth.

As you grow and get stronger, you can expect growing pains, but you have to remember that you are healing, and that is a process. Though trusting others is very important, you also have to be able to trust yourself. Trust your judgment, the healed you's intuition and not the one of old. Don't be afraid to cut toxicity off early before unhealthy attachments and bonds are formed. They will say that you are reacting because of your past, but you have to be strong, so you won't be manipulated to fall into the trap.

On this healing journey, I have lost a lot of people I thought were close to me and would be a part of my life for a long time. But as I began to grow, I knew I needed to be ok with letting the people go who did not need to be in my life. I was a "yes man" who would never use the word no. When people asked me to do anything, I always tried to figure out how to make it happen and please them. But when I healed, I knew that one of the keys to healing was saying no to others and yes to myself. I matter; my health matters, and having peace of mind matters more than pleasing others. We often hear people say that we need to be selfless, and I partially agree, but when it comes to being whole and protecting yourself from those who mentally drain you, you need to be very selfish. You have to learn to be a little selfish before you learn how to be selfless in a healthy way. When I talked to people struggling with depression and suicide, I heard them mention someone else during the process of them getting to that place. And what I found are people who are doing everything they can to build themselves up as they destroy another person with no regard.

I was driving Uber one day, and I arrived to pick this young lady up from a local college. When she got in my car, I noticed I was taking her to Methodist hospital. Though I could see what was going, on I decided to ask her where she was going. She said, "I am going to check in the mental hospital because I'm so depressed and on the verge of suicide."

"I'm sorry that you have hit a low point in your life and am glad to take you to go get help," I replied.

"Thank you," she said and began opening about her situation. "I am in an abusive relationship that I have kept from my parents for the past two years. He has beaten me and verbally abused me, and I didn't know how to break free. The other day he told me it was over, and now I'm lost without him. He was all I had."

I decided to pull no punches. I asked, "So, you are down and depressed because he dumped you after physically and verbally abusing you."

"Yes."

"Do you not see what is happening here?" "No," she said.

"He has given you the opportunity to find yourself and know your worth," I told her.

"He knows I struggle with depression and take meds. He told me that's why we fight, and he becomes abusive."

I said, "No, he hits and abuses you because he preys on your weakness, and he needs more help than you." When we arrived at the hospital, she walked in the doors, and I told her, "You got this, now go find yourself."

A few months later, I picked up the same young lady and asked her how she was doing? She told me she was doing well and was in counseling. I asked about her boyfriend, and she that they were still not together, but he wanted to get back with her.

"He hates the fact that I'm in counseling and getting the help that I need. He has spread rumors about me and caused our friends to turn their backs on me."

"Though it may hurt, it is a part of the process of walking in the new you. It's not about what he wants, but it's more about what you want and who you are becoming," I said. "The weak you would re-enter that relationship, but the strong you has somehow found the will to fight for you rather than fight for something that's unhealthy." She nodded her head in agreement and thanked me for the conversations we'd had prior to her being checked into the facility.

During my time at the juvenile detention center, I had many conversations with young men e affiliated with gangs. In many of our conversations, I would encourage them to move away and start all over. The main thing I would hear is, "I can't do that—I don't want my *opps* [competition] to feel like they have made me move." I often asked them if they were concerned about spending the rest of their lives in prison or ending up dead? And many of them would tell me they were ok with any of the above. They were so wrapped up in a life that promised them nothing and were willing to lose their lives for a reputation and a name. I witnessed it several times throughout my time there.

One day I went to a store close to where I lived, and I heard a young man yell my name.

"Ken! Aye, Ken!" As I turned around, he said, "You see me. I got a job now! I moved, and I'm not in them streets anymore. You remember that conversation we had, and you told me that if I was going to make it, I had to do the opposite of what everyone around me was doing. I thought about our conversation every night while in my cell."

I said, "Oh, yeah?"

"Yeah, man. I'm doing good." You could hear the sincerity in my voice when I told him how proud of him I was. But I remembered talking to him about his past, childhood, and some of the trauma he went through, so I asked him how that was going. He told me that he was getting the help he needed but that his mom and family were not happy with him talking to people about his problems. I remember looking him in his face and reminding him that it was not about what they wanted but about becoming a better man.

"You one-hundred percent right. I'm going to keep with it then," he said.

"Just remember, you are stronger than most people that come from where you come from."

His last words before we parted were, "One thing I've learned in this life is that even the closest people to me don't want to see me win."

What makes it hard when you are trying to better yourself is most of the people you are around—friendship, relationships, and family members are not at that same place. They are not ready to make those changes. You have to be willing to distance yourself, even if it's for a short time. You can't always expect them to celebrate with you because they are not in a place to celebrate their own lives. The longer you pursue being a better you, the more some will grow to accept the person you are becoming. But in the meantime, you better prepare yourself for the criticisms and gossip. *Who does he/she think she is now? I remember when they used to do this and that, now look at them.* Many people will get discouraged and fall back into their old ways because they don't get support from the people they desire the most. Again you are no good to them unless you are weak and easily influenced. And if you find yourself in a dark place again, they will be the ones to look you in your face and tell you *I told you so.*

When I left my neighborhood, I left with a suitcase of clothes and brought all the drama, trauma, and pain right along with me. And one day, after hitting rock bottom, I found myself in a car with my sisters, who were driving me back to the place I thought I'd overcome. When I came back to my neighborhood, I arrived with a suitcase and a $20 bill. I had nothing; I was homeless, with no car and no plan. When I returned home, I was the talk of the town. I specifically remember overhearing one conversation where the person said it looked like I did not have anything. He said I was broke and had done a whole bunch just to have nothing to show for it. Not once did someone say to me, "How can I help you get back on your feet?" What I heard was, "He is doing bad, and he just got out of a mental hospital." I was crushed, heartbroken, and ashamed of where I was.

After a few weeks of being in my old neighborhood, I woke up one morning and said this would be the last time I allowed my mental illness to get the best of me. I knew that it was time. The day I left, the same people who talked about me and my failures were still talking, even close relatives. But I made a decision to focus on myself regardless of what people thought. I was ready to make the changes. Though it was an uphill battle, I made it through the struggles.

When I moved to Illinois, I had nothing, but I found a way to overcome it through hard work and perseverance. I went from being broke and homeless to being an assistant superintendent at a juvenile detention center to finding one of the world's best therapists and being more mentally stable than I had ever been in my life. And most of all, I became a father to two beautiful girls, and in the midst of all this, I found my dream and my passion again. But if that does not make you happy, I am coming up on a decade since my last suicide attempt, and I have more reason to live now than I ever had before. Though I've hit some bumps in the road on this journey, I've found myself. I have grown to love myself and am at peace with who I am.

It does not matter what people say about you or how

unhappy they are with the healthy changes you have made. It does not matter who is not proud of you, slanders your name, or tries to steal your joy. For everything that I went through to live a life full of freedom, peace, and joy, it was all worth it. I am no longer a victim but an overcomer, and I did it all after being physically, sexually, and mentally abused. Yes, I have a mental illness, and I've developed mental toughness. I did not have the best life, but the rest of my life will be the best of my life. I am an overcomer.

CHAPTER FOURTEEN

REMAINING HEALED

If there is one promise that I can give you is that you will get hurt again. Even as I write this book, I am challenged to walk in the healed and new me. I have realized all the hard work that I have put in to get where I am made me unwilling to let anyone steal that from me. I continue to walk in healing by using the acronym,

H.E.A.L. I know that if I go outside of these guidelines for my life, I am on the way to a dark road again. I have worked too hard to go back. So, I focus on four main components: being **Honest** with myself, **Evaluating** my life, keeping **Accountability**, and letting go of painful **Experiences** a lot faster than I did in the past.

I smile all the time, and people used to ask me why I smiled so much? I used to tell them that I smile because I have been through enough in my life not to. That answer was so far from the truth. I used to smile because I wanted people to think that I was ok. When you smile, people assume that everything is going good in your life and shy away from asking you personal questions. But when I would go home and, alone or in one of many toxic relationships, I could not smile because reality would set in. I often wondered if I would smile for real or would that smile never have a true meaning. After going through the healing process, I now smile because I actually have joy and peace in my life. What changed? I have reached a point in my life where I can be honest with myself and those I am accountable to.

The first thing anyone who has experienced deep-rooted pain and trauma has to do is be honest with themselves. Hiding the real emotions and feelings does not make the issues go away. It just makes them become deep-rooted issues in our lives. When you get hurt by someone, it becomes a seed, and if it's not dealt with, it turns into a root and, from there, into a tree. It is much easier for us to deal with digging out a seed than for us to uproot a tree and its roots. And when it comes to mental and emotional health, those seeds are our feelings. Feelings are not bad things, but they become bad when we get stuck in them. Have you ever heard anyone say that you were in your feelings? Usually, what that means is that you took something way too personal that you should not have. Most of those incidents come from feeling trees left unacknowledged in our lives.

Though I have grown, I am still a very sensitive and

emotional person, and I get offended very easily. When I first started working at the JDC, there was one word that kids would use to get under my skin, and that was the B-word, pertaining to a female dog. Growing up in the inner-city, when someone called you the B-word, that meant they wanted to fight, and if you didn't fight or confront them, they would never stop messing with you. And growing up, you never wanted to be the B-word; it was not fun for you. The kids knew if they wanted to get me out of my character, they knew what to call me. After being called it over 1000 times, they noticed it did not bother me, so they stopped. I realized that I no longer had anything to prove, and they were not hurting me, but I was hurting myself by feeding into the negativity. But before I could get over it, I had to deal with the root of the problem.

My problem was, I had spent most of my life having to prove who I was to people. And I grew up never being able to defend myself from when I was a young kid, and I was never able to express how I felt unless it was anger and rage. So when I was in situations that trigger those emotions, I would take 1000 steps back in my life. If you hurt me with words, then I needed to hurt you with worse words, or we were going to have a physical altercation. All because I was afraid to admit when someone's words or actions were affecting me or hurting me.

Since healing, I have no problem with letting people know how I feel or how their actions are affecting me. I have learned to be honest with myself and others. Instead of running from tough moments, I have learned to face them that day or at least within 24 hours. My personal goal is I have five minutes to be upset and less than 24 hours to resolve an issue with people that are in my circle and that I am close to. This is because most of our hurt and trauma stems from people who are close to us or people who were supposed to protect us growing up. For the people who are not in my circle, I will address issues that need to be addressed, but if it does not add value to my life, I will usually ignore it and process it with the people in my circle. I do my best to make sure things don't grow a root. Learning to be honest with myself and how I feel is one of the key components to remaining healthy. Lies turn into truths when they are not addressed.

I find it amazing how we have a hard time expressing our opinions when it's what we feel. You or I should never be in a situation where we cannot healthily express ourselves. I have told myself that if my honest feelings are not voiced, then the situation has no real meaning to the problem or the person. Therefore if I allow myself to get hurt, it's a choice that I made to experience that hurt. No matter what I am feeling or what the other person has done in the conversation, there is value. Even if neither of us wants to be there, it is necessary if it's healthy and honest. Holding it in does nothing but create and foster negative emotions. And negativity is no good for anyone, but especially not good for those who already struggle mentally. So when you become healthy, you remain healthy by being honest with yourself and others.

When we are trying to remain healthy and are honest with ourselves, we constantly evaluate our lives. I find myself evaluating my life daily. I remember I had a conversation with someone, and I was expressing how I felt after I had just spent almost an hour listening to them express their feelings. I went home after the conversation feeling very defeated, but I felt as though I handled the incident correctly as I thought about it. But I continued to wrestle with it because I did not want them to not be a part of my life anymore. I sat down that night at the table and wrote down the pros and cons of not having a relationship with that person, and the cons outweighed the pros. That night I realized that I was not losing anything, and it would be detrimental to me remaining healthy. At that moment, evaluating became very beneficial. What I thought became true as weeks, months, and years went by.

When I was unhealthy, I never evaluated anything. I thought everything was good, and everyone had my best interests in mind. You learn over time that that is far from the truth. There are certain people who can smell a wounded person a mile away and prey on them to for their gain. That's why it's imperative to take inventory of our lives and not allow everyone in our circle. For me, I have set my circle to about five people that know everything about me and are who I rely on when I am needing to take inventory of the people around me. That does not mean I don't build relationships with others. It just means they aren't inner circle worthy.

Not only am I evaluating the people in my life, but I am also evaluating my moods, feelings, and emotions. When I am going through something, my first response is to isolate myself from the world. If my C-PTSD is being triggered, depending on the level, I schedule a therapy session, go for a walk or drive, hit the gym, or call one of my accountability partners. If that does not work, I usually will have my doctor up my medication dose until the symptoms decrease. For example, when my cousin died, I was having a tough time dealing with his death. Guilt set in, and I felt as though it was my fault. I increased my medication and my therapy sessions and made an appointment to talk to my circle about how I was feeling. By doing these steps, I was able to stop myself from going backward and continued moving in the right direction on the road to healing. Once my symptoms decreased, I was able to take get back on my normal routine.

I had a habit of running from tough situations and problems. I would deal with them by telling the person on the other end whatever it was they wanted to hear. But now I ask myself why and how after I've said yes to other people. I want to know why I said yes to them. Was it because I can actually do it, or because I wanted to get the situation done and over with? Then I ask myself, how is this going to affect me and my mental state? If I'm not honest, then it's only a matter of time before how I actually feel comes out. It's my way of protecting myself and others from any unneeded issues.

To remain healthy, I knew I needed to have some people in my life to hold me accountable. One of the hardest things for us who have been hurt or come from trauma is trusting others. I want to be the first person to tell you that contrary to popular belief, everyone is not bad. There are actually good people in this world and people who are willing to actually care about you and help you become whole. Though it's not something that happens overnight, you will have the opportunity to meet them over time. It is one of the key components of healing. We were never meant to walk through this life without other people in our lives. You did not get hurt alone, and you won't get through the hurt alone. Healing does not happen alone. We heal with people who are pushing our healing.

To be clear, what you are not looking for is someone willing to hold others accountable but unwilling to hold themselves accountable. If they are challenging you in an area, it should be someone who has or is growing in that area. They need to be someone who will help you grow even when you hit your lowest points. It has to be a judgment-free zone. I believed that this should not be a family member, but I realized that we all come from different backgrounds. Some of you come from good and healthy backgrounds, so you could have a healthy family member be that person for you. If you come from a trauma-based family, then it is very unhealthy for you to have those family members hold you accountable.

Accountability only works if you are willing, being honest with the people holding you accountable. You can't get mad with them if you aren't being upfront with what you are feeling. They are there to walk with you through the ups and downs and make sure you are putting the time and energy into working through the downs. It is unfair that you only go to them when you are at your low moments. Healthy accountability happens at all different levels of your battles. I remember walking into a counselor's office and asking them to fix a broken relationship. When we both walked into the office, we knew that the relationship was over and was beyond repair, or should I say we were past working on our issues with one another. For months, we wasted that counselor's time because we did not practice or work on any strategies presented to us. We wanted someone to tell us what we already knew. We were not trying to heal. To heal or remain in the healing process, you will need accountability. You will have to find someone to start with. I found it easy to start building accountability with my therapist, and I could branch out from there.

You will have some low moments, and that's what they are there for to help lift you up and keep you on track. The more you are in groups of accountabilities, the less likely the lows will move you backward.

The final thing I do to remain in a healed state of mind is that I have learned to let things go a lot faster. Many of my hurtful times and moments followed me for years. As I shared in earlier chapters, I was afraid to let go. As I began to evaluate my life and how many things I'd lost during the process, I learned carrying the pain was not worth it. I am not saying they did not affect me. What I am saying is I allowed them to affect me longer than I should have. Now when I face tough moments, I process them quickly and let them go. You notice I did not say blow them off but process them first. Processing is learning what you need to learn from it and keep it moving forward.

This does not mean you make excuses for what others say or do, giving situations a shoulder shrug. No, you take a full inventory of what happened, process how to deal with it, and let it go, which sometimes requires you to let them go. I was in a meeting once, and my character was being attacked with many accusations, including my mental illness. Their whole goal was to rip me into shreds and make me lose my credibility. A few months later, I began to open myself up to a relationship with them, but I was healthier, and I realized that no accountability was taken for their actions. Instead, they wanted to ignore what transpired. I left that day and realized I had to let them go because they would do it to me again. A person with no regard for their actions towards you needs to be let go.

When I forgave my mom that day, it felt as if an eighteen-wheeler truck had been lifted off my heart. That was an amazing feeling and was the beginning of my healing journey. Any issue that has caused you to feel weighed down and not yourself needs to be lifted, and that only happens when you let things go. Small weights turn into heavy weights, and we have no room in our lives for either. In order to walk free, we have to lose the offenses that become boulders and blinders in our lives.

I was not born with a mental illness. It came from traumatic experiences in my life. Now that I have overcome those situations, I want to continue to walk in the freedom I know. Because I have faced so many challenges, been suicidal, battled depression, and been diagnosed with C-PTSD, I have to work hard every day to live my life in a healed state. It took me twenty-plus years to get to this point in my life. The acronym H.E.A.L. can be used for people who don't have mental illnesses and the people who have loved ones or friends walking through life struggling mentally. Your freedom will be determined by you. You are not the first, nor will you be the last, to battle your mental illness. But you will always have a choice to land on the end of the spectrum where you're controlled by it or the one who learns how to cope and help others heal. The people who heal will be the ones to help mental illness become less taboo. The more of us that heal, the more normal our struggle will become. Pain, trauma and suicide did not defeat me because I overcame! From adolescent trauma to a life of adult brokenness, I have learned to make C-PTSD look manageable, and so can you!